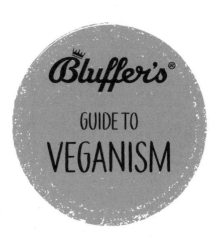

Bluffer's®

GUIDE TO
VEGANISM

D0620582

BORIS STARLING

A CIP Catalogue record for this book
is available from the British Library.

ISBN: 978 1 78521 670 1

Library of Congress control no. 2019948727

Published by Haynes Publishing,
Sparkford, Yeovil, Somerset BA22 7JJ, UK
Tel: 01963 440635
Int. tel: +44 1963 440635
Website: www.haynes.com

Printed in Malaysia.

Bluffer's Guide®, Bluffer's® and Bluff Your Way®
are registered trademarks.

Series Editor: David Allsop.

CONTENTS

'There is nothing so powerful as an idea whose time has come.'

Victor Hugo

COOL BEANS: WHY VEGANISM IS SUDDENLY HOT

Welcome to *The Bluffer's Guide To Veganism*. Veganism is on the rise, and unlike other alternative diets and ways of living, it seems here to stay. In fact, the word 'vegan' has been around since 1944, and the practice of abstaining from eating or wearing any animal products even longer (*see* pages 63/64).

The number of vegans in the UK quadrupled from 150,000 to 600,000 between 2014 and 2018.[1] Sign-ups for the Veganuary campaign – where people go vegan for the month of January – nearly doubled in 2019, with 250,000 people joining – as much as the three previous years combined. The UK launched more vegan products

1 Ipsos Mori survey commissioned by the Vegan Society, 2018.

than any nation in 2018,[2] and the country's meat-free market (which is garnering increasing attention and investment from traditional food giants among others) is estimated to grow from £559m in 2016 to £658m in 2021.[3]

Sooner or later, therefore, and especially given the importance of food in our daily lives, the bluffer will be called into action on the topic of veganism. The guiding principle of bluffing, and the raison d'être of the *Bluffer's Guides* (now entering their fifth decade of imparting instant wit and wisdom) is that a little knowledge is a desirable thing. Since that is all most of us are ever going to have anyway, we might as well get to know how to spread it thinly but effectively (like Marmite, itself an excellent vegan staple).

Careful manipulation of some rudimentary facts will help you bluff your way through with a reasonable degree of nonchalance. This is especially important in these heady days of instant online information. When everyone has Google literally at their fingertips, failure to polish your bluffing techniques will leave you at a social and professional disadvantage.

This book is therefore not a 'how to' guide, but rather a 'how to pretend you know how to' guide. (There is a subtle distinction.) As our series strapline reads: 'It's not what you know, it's what they think you know.' So come in hard, drop some esoteric facts, make a few opaque allusions, and with any luck your interlocutors will

2 Nielsen Scantrack, 2018.
3 Mintel 'Meat Free Food' report, May 2017.

think you have the kind of inside knowledge usually confined to the most erudite of historians. If in doubt, ask yourself: What would Bruce Willis do? He'd bluff hard. He'd bluff harder. And when all else failed, he'd bluff hard with a vengeance.

Be like Bruce.

(Bruce isn't a vegan himself, but he spends a lot of time in Hollywood, where there *are* loads of vegans, so that'll do for us. Tenuous connections are one of the bluffer's raisons d'etre, after all.)

VEGANALYSIS

So, where to start? Call us bluffers old traditionalists, but how about the basics? What is veganism, and how does it differ from vegetarianism?

Vegans eat no animal products: not just animal flesh or parts, but anything which comes from animals at all. No meat, no poultry, no fish or shellfish, no eggs, no dairy products, no insects, no honey, no animal protein such as rennet or gelatine, and no stock or fats which derive from animals.

In contrast, vegetarians won't eat animal flesh, but may eat products which come from animals. Ovo-lacto vegetarians eat eggs and dairy products; ovo vegetarians eat eggs but not dairy; and lacto vegetarians eat dairy but not milk. Pescatarians, who eat fish and other seafood but not meat, are sometimes considered vegetarians even though technically they are not so. (Such pedantry is of course catnip to the bluffer.) And then there are flexitarians, who declare themselves usually, but not always, vegetarian (i.e. when they wake up with an emperor-sized hangover on Saturday morning, it's a full English for breakfast followed by a lunchtime Big Mac, principles be (temporarily) damned).

But veganism is not just a question of diet. The Vegan Society defines veganism as 'a way of living which seeks to exclude, as far as is possible and practicable, all forms of exploitation of, and cruelty to, animals for food, clothing or any other purpose'. To this extent it is a moral position, even a philosophy. Strict vegans avoid wearing clothes made from animal skin or by-products – leather, suede, wool, silk and so on. They eschew products which have been tested on animals or contain animal parts (such as soaps and candles made partially from tallow), and oppose the use of animals in entertainment (circuses, carriage rides, zoos, marine parks).

As any hardened bluffer knows, correlation does not necessarily equal causation (a phrase which the bluffer should deploy judiciously but effectively).

As for why veganism is suddenly so popular: well, there are several reasons. Most vegans, whether newly-converted or long-established, cite one or more of three main factors for their decision: animal welfare, personal health and environmental concerns (see *Peas of Mind*,

Couch Potato and *Rocket Science* chapters respectively). But these three areas of concern have been around for years, so they do not by themselves explain the sudden, almost exponential growth of the vegan movement over the past few years.

What *is* new, and what has been and continues to be a huge driver of the shift towards veganism, is social media. It's no accident that the growth in veganism mirrors almost exactly the rise of social media. As any hardened bluffer knows, correlation does not necessarily equal causation (a phrase which the bluffer should deploy judiciously but effectively), but in this case correlation does most definitely equal causation.

A few decades ago, vegans were mocked and feared in equal measures – as hippies or punks whose eating habits were an integral part of their undesirably counter-cultural lifestyles, or as animal rights radicals taking aggressive and often eye-catching direct action against perceived transgressors. But social media has allowed veganism to rebrand itself as cool, trendy, healthy, caring and aspirational, all of which greatly appeal to the younger demographic most active in social networking – and it is this demographic who are most readily making the switch to veganism.

'The shift toward plant-based foods is being driven by millennials,' said *Forbes* magazine in 2017. (If you're a *Daily Telegraph* reader, you may wish to substitute the words 'Generation Snowflake' for 'millennials'.) What matters to young people will matter on social media. After all, that's where they get most of their information these days. They don't even have to be looking for vegan information: it will be pushed towards them by the relentless algorithms (as opposed to the rather less relentless Al Gore), often while they're browsing for something completely different.

Social media has allowed veganism to rebrand itself as cool, trendy, healthy, caring and aspirational, all of which greatly appeal to the younger demographic most active in social networking.

If you've ever sat in a restaurant and watched someone on another table climb on their chair to get a better smartphone picture of their dish, and if you've ever muttered 'For the love of God, just eat the damn food' while observing this performance, you'll know that few things appeal to Instagram or Pinterest aficionados as much as food pictures. Vegan food is no different. Artfully arranged and well photographed, it can appear every bit as appealing as non-vegan food – and if you mentally substituted the word 'normal' for 'non-vegan' there, you're probably in the majority, at least for now (*see* the chapter *Romaines to be Seen* for a look at a future where veganism is normal and carnism, meat-eating, is the weirdo minority interest).

Add to this the role of celebrities and 'influencers' in promoting veganism online (yes, the bluffer should know that being an online 'influencer' is a real job, and that sound you can hear is a legion of long-deceased school careers officers spinning in their graves; no, being an online influencer almost certainly not what Dale Carnegie had in mind when he wrote *How To Win Friends and Influence People*), and the bluffer can wax lyrical about the mushroom effect of trends and tribes in a world where people spend an ever-increasing proportion of their lives online. 'If you look back even five years ago,' says Edward Bergen, global food and drink analyst at market research company Mintel, 'veganism was probably considered a bit of a joke. [But now] consumers listen to celebrities and influencers about what they do.'

There are vegan cooks on YouTube, vegan groups on Facebook and vegan documentaries on Netflix, all accessible at the click of a button. Kip Andersen, co-director of the documentary *Cowspiracy*, says that 'People feel empowered, it doesn't feel like a sacrifice. That's a huge shift. Whereas before veganism may have been viewed like you were giving up something, now it's been reframed as what you gain: you gain health, you gain a greater sense of living in bounds with your values, you gain all the environmental benefits.'

And, since no online trend is complete without a healthy dose of controversy, the bluffer can point out that Google search volumes for 'veganism' are outpacing those for 'vegetarianism' by almost three to one, and one of the reasons for this is that veganism attracts more naysayers than vegetarianism. It's seen as more hardcore and less forgiving and/or practical, which allows opponents to weigh in more heavily than they would do on vegetarianism, which is less proscriptive and therefore less controversial.

Veganism in particular straddles quite a few separate touchpaper topics: health, environment, ethics, socio-economics and politics. Given that any one of these can spark off intense and heated debate/arguments/fights, the combination of several puts veganism firmly in the realm of lighting blue touchpaper and retiring. (If the bluffer comes across anyone who still doubts the role of social media in creating and reinforcing tribes, the words 'Brexit' and 'Trump' should spring unbidden to mind. Reasoned and moderate arguments tend to get drowned out by the extremists, who take any attack on their beliefs as an attack on themselves, double down on their arguments, and demand of others that they are either with them or against them.)

The particularly confident bluffer will go a step further by referring to 'an assemblage of several actors and platforms, with discursive and lifestyle political consumerism and their interplay characterising the current building of new images and communities'.

William Sitwell, former editor of *Waitrose Food* magazine, was obliged to step down in October 2018 after suggesting 'a series on killing vegans, one by one. Ways to trap them? How to interrogate them properly? Expose their hypocrisy? Force-feed them meat? Make them eat steak and drink red wine?' in an e-mail to vegan journalist Selene Nelson. Your mileage may vary on whether or not he should have lost his job over the issue, and/or whether Nelson was right to make public the contents of a private e-mail, but the bluffer should confidently opine that what *does* seem beyond doubt is that, had this taken place even two or three years earlier, let alone five or ten, the whole incident would likely have passed off without much hoopla.

There are therefore several factors at play in the rise of veganism – or, as the bluffer should put it, 'several congruent, concurrent and yet discrete factors'. The particularly confident bluffer (and let's face it, should there be any other kind?) will go a step further by referring to 'an assemblage of several actors and platforms, with discursive and lifestyle political consumerism and their interplay characterising the current building of new images and communities'. (No, me neither, but it sounds good, and for the bluffer that is half the battle won before it's even started.)

VEGANATOMY

The Bluffer's Guide to Veganism is divided into several sections.

Bean There looks at the history of veganism. *Peas of*

Mind, Couch Potato and *Rocket Science* examine the three main reasons for people becoming vegan as outlined above: animal rights, health and the environment respectively. *Salad Gold* outlines the mainstays of a vegan diet, and *Kale of Duty* those of a wider vegan lifestyle. *Turning over a New Leaf* looks at how best to make the transition to veganism. *Know Your Onions* sets up and knocks down some of the most common objections to veganism (a quintessentially bluffer's chapter, this one). *I Herb It Through the Grapevine* takes you on a whistlestop vegan tour of the world, *Sowing Oats* looks at veganism and sex, and *Romaines to be Seen* deals with the future of veganism. Finally, *Amaizing Grace* is a personal (and perhaps slightly unexpected) conclusion, before the *Alphabet Black Bean Soup* of the glossary.

Enjoy, and happy bluffing.

BEAN THERE: THE HISTORY OF VEGANISM

'The day has been, I am sad to say in many places it is not yet past, in which the greater part of the species, under the denomination of slaves, have been treated by the law exactly upon the same footing, as, in England for example, the inferior races of animals are still. The day may come when the rest of the animal creation may acquire those rights which never could have been withholden from them but by the hand of tyranny. The French have already discovered that the blackness of the skin is no reason a human being should be abandoned without redress to the caprice of a tormentor. It may one day come to be recognised that the number of the legs, the villosity of the skin, or the termination of the os sacrum are reasons equally insufficient for abandoning a sensitive being to the same fate. What else is it that should trace the insuperable line? Is it the faculty of reason or perhaps the faculty of discourse? But a full-grown horse or dog, is beyond comparison a more rational, as well as a more conversable animal, than an infant of a day or a

week or even a month, old. But suppose the case were otherwise, what would it avail? The question is not, "can they reason?", nor "can they talk?", but rather "can they suffer?"'

Introduction to the Principles of Morals and Legislation, *Jeremy Bentham, 1789*

Veganism's sudden recent popularity should not obscure the fact that, one way or another, it is a practice which goes back many millennia. Diets in the Neolithic period (the end of the Stone Age, around 12,000 years ago, an era in which quite a few modern-day attitudes seem mired if newspaper online comment sections are anything to go by) were mainly plant-based, with meat scavenged and consumed relatively rarely (either as part of ceremonial feasting or through necessity when staple crops were in short supply).

Veganism appears in several major religions. In the Bible, the Garden of Eden was a vegan paradise. 'And God said, Behold, I have given you every herb bearing seed, which is upon the face of all the earth, and every tree, in the which is the fruit of a tree yielding seed; to you it shall be for meat.'[4] (The bluffer should always have a biblical quote or several to hand.)

The three *ahisma* (non-violence) religions of the Indian subcontinent, Hinduism, Buddhism and Jainism, all promote plant-based diets; indeed, Jains try to avoid even accidental harm to insects by wearing muslin cloths over their mouths and brushing the ground in front of themselves as they walk.

4   Genesis chapter 1, verse 29.

Both ancient Rome and ancient Greece (again, these are bluffers' staples) knew of veganism. The Roman poet Ovid and playwright Seneca the Younger followed plant-based diets, as did the Greek philosopher Plutarch and mathematician Pythagoras. Eudoxus of Cnidus, a student of Plato, wrote that 'Pythagoras was distinguished by such purity and so avoided killing and killers that he not only abstained from animal foods, but even kept his distance from cooks and hunters.' (We can therefore conclude that he almost certainly never appeared on *The Great Athenian Bake-Off*.)

Being overweight was a source of pride rather than shame: it meant that one could afford the kind of foods which made one fat, and in the days before mass processing of food that as often as not meant meat.

For much of history, of course, meat and its consumption have been one of the great markers of wealth. Being overweight was a source of pride rather than shame: it meant that one could afford the kind of foods which made one fat, and in the days before mass processing of food that as often as not meant meat.

But that wasn't to say that this way of life was universally seen as desirable. Bentham was one of the earliest proponents of animal rights, and, as the opening quote of this section shows, was concerned above all with the imperative to minimise or eliminate animal suffering – a stance which would surely have seen him horrified by today's factory farming practices (*see* the chapter *Peas of Mind*).

'*I never have seen, nor ever can see, any objection to the putting of dogs and other inferior animals to pain, in the way of medical experiment, when that experiment has a determinate object, beneficial to mankind, accompanied with a fair prospect of the accomplishment of it. But I have a decided and insuperable objection to the putting of them to pain without any such view. To my apprehension, every act by which, without prospect of preponderant good, pain is knowingly and willingly produced in any being what-so-ever, is an act of cruelty; and, like other bad habits, the more the correspondent habit is indulged in, the stronger it grows, and the more frequently productive of its bad fruit. I am unable to comprehend how it should be, that to him to whom it is a matter of amusement to see a dog or a horse suffer, it should not be a matter of like amusement to see a man suffer; seeing, as I do, how much more morality as well as intelligence, an adult quadruped of those and many other species has in him, than any biped has for some months after he has been brought into existence; nor does it appear to me how it should be, that a person to whom the production of pain, either in the one or in the other instance, is a source of amusement, would scruple to give himself that amusement when he could do so under an assurance of impunity.*'[5] (If you can remember all that,

5   Letter to the editor of the *Morning Chronicle*, 1825.

there's a future for you on game shows, in GCHQ, or both.)

Around the same era, the poet Percy Bysshe Shelley's 1813 *A Vindication of Natural Diet* advocated 'abstinence from animal food and spirituous liquors'. (Then again he did describe coffee-shop proprietor Mrs Miggins as 'lovelorn ecstasy', at least according to series 3 of *Blackadder*.)

THE VEGETARIAN SPECTRUM

The UK Vegetarian Society was founded in 1847, and over the following decades positioned itself at the more moderate end of the vegetarian spectrum. In 1884, *The Medical Times and Gazette* in London said that 'there are

---

It was not until November 1944 – when, of course, meat was being severely rationed during the Second World War and plant-based diets were both necessary and patriotic ('Dig for Victory') – that the name 'vegan' came into existence.

---

two kinds of vegetarians – one an extreme form, the members of which eat no animal food products what-so-ever; and a less extreme sect, who do not object to eggs, milk, or fish. The Vegetarian Society ... belongs to the latter more moderate division.' (This *Bluffer's Guide* is now seriously considering a campaign to restore the word 'whatsoever' to its former spelling, 'what-so-ever', as shown here, and perhaps even expanding this campaign to encompass 'none-the-less' and 'not-with-standing' too.)

Yet there was still no official name given to these dangerous, extreme radicals who abjured all animal products and clearly put the wind up the genteel Victorian vegetarians. Were there glowering stand-offs over afternoon tea, with the cucumber sandwich die-hards sneering at those who dared essay the egg and cress? In fact, it was not until November 1944 – when, of course, meat was being severely rationed during the Second World War and plant-based diets were both necessary and patriotic ('Dig for Victory') – that the name 'vegan' came into existence.

It was coined by Donald Watson, secretary of the Vegetarian Society's Leicester branch, who had decided to become what he hadn't yet named after witnessing the death of a pig on his uncle's farm. 'I decided that farms, and uncles, had to be reassessed.' When his request that the Vegetarian Society include in its magazine a section about non-dairy diets was turned down, he set up a breakaway newsletter called *The Vegan News* – 'vegan' being a word he'd invented himself from the first three and last two letters of 'vegetarian' because that signified 'the beginning and end of vegetarian'.

Watson asked his readers whether they could think of a better word, and several alternatives were suggested. Among them were:

- 'allvega' (which looks very like the annoying selection of Scrabble tiles you sometimes find on your slate which almost make several words of decent length but none of them exactly)
- 'beaumangeur' (the lesser-known confrère of Beau Geste)
- 'benevore' (nothing to do with American indie band Bon Iver)
- 'dairyban' (a piece of Newspeak which Orwell excised before the final draft of *Nineteen Eighty-Four*)
- 'neo-vegetarian' (just dull)
- 'sanivore' (surely a trade name waiting to happen for an ointment designed to cure a minor but excruciatingly embarrassing medical complaint)
- and 'vitan' (which turns out to be an unlovely suburb of the Romanian capital Bucharest).

Perhaps unsurprisingly, none of these really caught on, so 'vegan' it was and 'vegan' it's stayed. But you will get plenty of bonus bluffer points if you drop a well-timed 'benevore' or 'dairyban' into conversation.

Watson himself lived to the grand old age of 95. His funeral, he liked to say, would be a big one no matter how long he lived. 'There'll be a smattering of people, but there'll also be the spirits of all the animals I've never eaten.' World Vegan Day is held every 1 November to mark his founding of the Vegan Society.

(Leicester's other great contribution to veganism is, of course, Walker's Crisps. The humble pie which Leicester City football club forced every other Premiership club to eat during their triumphal campaign of 2015–16 wasn't vegan, including as it did ingredients which obliged its recipients to also eat:

(a) crow
(b) their hats
(c) their words
(d) their shorts
(e) their hearts out.)

NICHE NOTIONS

For much of the period since the founding of the Vegan Society, veganism was a niche interest both in the UK and the US, and – as mentioned in *Cool Beans* – largely associated with the counterculture: anarchists, hippies and punks. People for the Ethical Treatment of Animals (PETA) was founded in 1980, and their modus operandi – eye-catching radical protests – brought them much press (and police) attention, but did little to really change wider public attitudes towards eating animals.

Only now, with social media allowing people to feel themselves charmed into supporting veganism rather than bludgeoned into it, are things really changing. (This is an ideal juncture for the bluffer to muse on the manner in which public attitudes towards minority rights have been changed over the years: the tactics used by the suffragettes in Edwardian times, for instance, were very different to those used by gay activists in the 1980s. By throwing this question open to the floor, the bluffer can portray themself as a person of great and thoughtful hinterland.)

PEAS OF MIND (REASONS TO BE VEGAN, PART 1)

THE ETHICS OF ANIMAL WELFARE

Every year in the UK an estimated 950m birds, 80m fish, 10m pigs and 2.5m cows are slaughtered for human consumption.[6] Vegans object to three aspects of this: the simple fact of the slaughter itself, the unnecessarily cruel manner in which the slaughter is often carried out, and the conditions in which the animals are forced to live while awaiting their inevitable and premature end.

Animal welfare is consistently cited as the number one reason for people becoming vegan. For vegans this is, quite literally, a matter of life and death.

At this point, the bluffer should drop in the concept

6   Humane Slaughter Association.

of the 'schema'. A schema is a pattern of thought, a cognitive framework which helps us organise and interpret categories of information and the relationships between them. We have schemata (bonus bluffer points for the correct use of the plural there) for pretty much every subject we come across, including animals. 'An animal can be classified as prey, predator, pest, pet, or food,' says the social psychologist Melanie Joy. 'How we classify an animal, in turn, determines how we relate to it – whether we hunt it, flee from it, exterminate it, love it, or eat it. When it comes to meat, most animals are either food, or not food. In other words, we have a schema that classifies animals as edible or inedible.

'And within the edible–inedible dichotomy, we have a number of other category pairs. For example, we eat domesticated rather than wild animals, and herbivores rather than omnivores or carnivores. Most people won't eat animals that they deem intelligent (dolphins), but regularly consume those they believe are not very smart (cows and chickens). [They] avoid eating animals that they perceive as cute (rabbits) and instead eat animals that they consider less attractive (turkeys).

'One reason we have such different perceptions of beef and dog meat is because we view cows and dogs very differently. The most frequent – and often the only – contact we have with cows is when we eat (or wear) them. But our relationship with dogs is, in many ways, not terribly different from our relationship with people. We call them by their names. We say goodbye when we leave and greet them when we return. We share our beds with them. We play with them. We buy them gifts. We take them to the doctor when they're sick and may spend thousands of dollars on their treatment. We bury them when they pass away. They make us laugh; they make us cry. They are our helpers, our friends, our family. We love them. We love dogs and eat cows not because dogs and cows are fundamentally different – cows, like dogs, have feelings, preferences, and consciousness – but because our perception of them is different. And, consequently, our perception of their meat is different as well.'[7]

'An animal can be classified as prey, predator, pest, pet, or food. How we classify an animal, in turn, determines how we relate to it – whether we hunt it, flee from it, exterminate it, love it, or eat it.'

This schema is so well entrenched in society – rather like the concept of eating meat itself – that it passes unchallenged most of the time. And when it *is* challenged, the usual response (as is often the case with schemata) is to discount the challenging information rather than use it to change the schema. For example, the vast majority of Westerners find the Asian habit of eating dog meat to be cruel, repulsive and unfathomable, and therefore react either with incomprehension or mockery. As an

7   *Why We Love Dogs, Eat Pigs, and Wear Cows*, 2009.

example of the latter, Manchester United fans greeted South Korean footballer Park Ji-Sung's 2005 arrival at their club with the terrace chants 'He shoots, he scores/ he eats your Labradors' and, to the tune of *Lord of the Dance*, 'Park, Park, wherever you may be/they eat dogs in your home country.' (Being able to quote the Bible, Jeremy Bentham and Manchester United fans in the same breath is Bluffer's 101, obviously.)

In other words they, like most of us, rationalised this habit as something belonging to an alien culture and therefore outside our usual social mores, rather than considering that perhaps the eating of dog meat is logically consistent with an omnivorous diet (which, in purely nutritional terms, it is). 'Despite the fact that it's perfectly legal in 44 [of America's 50] states, eating "man's best friend" is as taboo as a man eating his best friend,' says the American writer Jonathan Safran Foer. 'There are laws in all fifty states prohibiting cruelty to animals. The laws vary from state to state, but not in one respect: in every state, the legislation that prohibits cruelty to animals exempts animals destined for human consumption. In every single one of the 50 states, if you are raising an animal for meat, for milk, or for eggs, you can without restriction subject that animal to conditions which, if you did that to a dog or a cat, would land you in jail.'[8]

A similar situation applies in most developed countries, including the UK. 'The standard operating procedures in the industry are not designed to be cruel. That is not their goal or their intent. They are designed to be cost effective. But if it turns out that it is cost effective

8   *Eating Animals*, 2009.

to confine animals in conditions that actually resemble Auschwitz or Dachau, then that's what will happen.'[9]

Even if every factory farm threw its gates open to anyone and everyone, many people still wouldn't want to know. There's too much else in everyday life to worry about – Brexit, the mortgage, *Love Island*. ...

That these conditions are not better known is due to a combination of factors. Few, if any, factory farms allow reporters inside (in fairness, as the bluffer should point out, this is not confined to agriculture: few large companies in any sector do, as much for commercially sensitive reasons as anything more nefarious), which means that activists and journalists need to rely on dangerous and difficult undercover investigations. Large agricultural firms (BigAg) are just as adept as their BigPharma/BigOil counterparts at lobbying governments to maintain their economic and legislative advantages.

And even if they weren't, and even if every factory farm threw its gates open to anyone and everyone, many people still wouldn't want to know. There's too much else in everyday life to worry about – Brexit, the mortgage, *Love Island* – and it's cognitively hard for the

9   Joy, ibid.

human mind to process the individual cost of such large-scale suffering, be it animals or humans. As Stalin is reported to have said, 'A single death is a tragedy. A million deaths is a statistic.' (Consider that the European refugee crisis began in 2010, but a concerted international response didn't take place until the 2015 photograph of three-year-old Alan Kurdi's dead body on a Turkish beach prompted public outrage.)

Factory farms now account for the vast majority of animals destined for slaughter. 'We shouldn't kid ourselves about the number of ethical eating options available to most of us. There isn't enough non-factory chicken produced in America to feed the population of Staten Island, and not enough non-factory pork to serve New York City, let alone the country. Ethical meat is a promissory note, not a reality. Any ethical-meat advocate who is serious is going to be eating a lot of vegetarian fare. For me, factory farming is wrong not because it produces meat, but because it robs every animal of every shred of happiness.'[10]

ANIMAL FACTORIES

In the interests of this book not ending up the same length as *War And Peace*, we will look at only four of the most common categories of slaughtered animal: chickens, cows, pigs and fish. Be aware, this will make uncomfortable reading – but at the core of successful bluffing is an acknowledgement that certain unavoidable and unpalatable realities will sometimes have to be confronted

10 Foer, ibid.

if bluffers want to pass as experts in any subject, especially one as emotive and contentious as animal welfare.

You will need to be familiar with these arguments if you are to be taken as an expert in veganism, which – after all – is your goal. You don't have to take a position on factory farming because, lest it be forgotten, you're a bluffer. You just have to give the impression that you have considered all the arguments, and are having some difficulty in making those defending the mass slaughter of animals stand up.

As you rehearse some of the following vegan claims, you might accompany them with a disbelieving shake of the head and sharp intake of breath. Don't worry – if you have an enquiring mind and an ounce of compassion this will come with relative ease, and you might look at what's on your plate and in your wardrobe with a renewed focus.

CHICKENS

Chickens can be great characters. They're active and inquisitive, forever foraging and exploring. They dust-bathe the way we will have a bath, and chat endlessly to each other. Watch any group of chickens in a run where they are given adequate space and decent shelter and nutrition, and it won't be long before you can distinguish them not just by looks but also by personality.

All of that counts for nothing when it comes to large-scale commercial rearing. The bluffer should know that chickens are divided into two categories: broilers (to be eaten), and layers (to produce eggs). They have been bred in such radically different ways that they are now practically genetically distinct from each other.

Around 90% of broilers in the UK are raised in vast sheds, often windowless, which can house up to 50,000 chickens each.[11] In natural conditions, broilers could live for ten years, often more. In factory farms, they'll be lucky to make it to seven weeks, not just because that ensures a constant turnover and supply of new birds, but also because they're pumped full of growth-promoting drugs. The human equivalent would be a 25-stone two-year-old. No, that's not a misprint. (This kind of factbomb is more of a depth charge when used by the skilful bluffer. Dropped in at the right moment, it should bring any conversation to a juddering if temporary halt.)

This comes, of course, at a great cost to the chickens' health. Their legs often twist and break under the strain of carrying all that weight. If they fall to the floor and can't get up, they suffer skin burns from the ammonia in the litter all over the ground. Heart failure is common. Dead birds are often simply left where they've fallen until the time comes to take the live ones off to slaughter. The cramped conditions and overcrowding mean that the chickens can't behave as they would naturally – foraging, exploring, nesting, dust-bathing – so they lash out, which in turn means that they're debeaked (by a hot blade, without anaesthesia, at birth) to prevent them damaging each other.

Layers (battery hens) are treated slightly better (though the bluffer should very much emphasise the word 'slightly': that is, not enough to make any meaningful difference, and still cruelly by any

11 Animal Aid factsheet, 2019.

reasonable definition of the word). They usually live for around 18 months before being slaughtered (i.e. when their egg-laying capacity begins to diminish), and most spend the entirety of those lives in cages, with each hen allocated an iPad's worth of space. (The original battery cages were banned in the UK in 2012, but the new 'colony cages' offer only marginally more space.) They exist under artificial lights designed to encourage them to lay as many eggs as possible, and many suffer broken legs and wings when calcium is extracted from their bones and placed in their diet to help make eggshells.

Of course, 50% of all newborn chicks are males, who can't lay eggs, whose meat isn't nearly as good as the females', and who are all in all therefore rather surplus to requirements. What happens to them? Exactly what you might think. Every year, 40m day-old chicks are killed in the UK, either gassed or thrown into a macerator. They're supposed to be stunned unconscious in a water bath first, but it doesn't always happen that way, to say the least.

All chickens of whatever age, broilers and layers alike, are supposed to be stunned first before slaughter. Adult chickens are usually hung upside down and have their necks cut post-stunning, but when the stunning fails the cutting is done anyway while the chickens are conscious, and it can take several minutes for the birds to bleed out and die.

This method of slaughter applies whether the chickens have been kept in factory farms or as 'free range'. It's a little like priority boarding on a budget airline flight: no matter how fancy the appellation, you end up in the same place. In any case, the difference between factory and free range can be moot. If the words 'free range' conjure up vistas of happy hens roaming vast swathes of ground under bright sunshine – well, to don the hat of the cynical bluffer (a subspecies of *bluffus bluffus*), that's marketing for you, free and easy with the facts but fast and loose with the truth. Free range has to have some kind of outdoor facility, but in many cases that's as far as it goes.

The official government guidelines issued by the Department for the Environment, Food and Rural Affairs (DEFRA) state that *'Sufficient housing should be available to the birds at all times. … Birds should be encouraged to use the outdoor area. Provision of adequate, suitable and properly managed vegetation, overhead cover forming corridors leading out from the house and distributed around the range and a supply of fresh water away from the house, will help induce the birds to range. Feed should not be routinely provided outdoors.'*

In other words, there are no concrete stipulations at all about how often birds should be outside, nor the size of any outside run, nor the parameters of access to the outside. There are lots of suggestions and guidelines, but the actual conditions are pretty much entirely at the producer's discretion.

(The US Department of Agriculture's guidelines are even flimsier: literally the sole criterion for free range is that 'producers must demonstrate that the poultry has been allowed access to the outside'. That is, a tiny patch of ground accessible only by a single small door in a vast warehouse can technically count as being 'free range'. And even with lots of doors, many hens would never get to go outside: hens are territorial, and stronger birds will not let weaker birds cross their space.)

COWS

The bluffer should go big on the similarities between chickens and cows (when it comes to their role in the human food chain, that is, not necessarily to look at).

Like chickens, cows have distinct personalities and thrive on social interaction. Like chickens, cows are increasingly divided into two categories, in this case beef and milk. Like chickens, male cows are deemed much less important and useful than female ones. And, like chickens, cows reared in cramped conditions, pumped full of drugs and killed long before the end of their natural lifespan are given little or no chance to develop normal behavioural patterns.

With cows, however, there's one crucial difference. They're viviparous rather than oviparous (both useful bluffer's words), and the bond between mother and child is stronger than between chicken and chick. Left to her own devices, a cow will take herself away from the herd when she's about to give birth, return once she's ready to introduce the newborn to the herd, and then suckle her calf for between nine and 12 months.

In factory dairy farming (usually with specifically bred Holstein or Friesian cows), none of this happens. The calf is taken away from the mother within hours to prevent it from drinking her milk, which will instead go to the dairy industry. Female calves are kept in individual hutches far from their mothers, a separation which is traumatic for both of them: they often call out to each other for hours or even days on end. Under EU law the calves must be put into groups after eight weeks, but by then the nurturing bond is damaged beyond repair.

Then the cycle begins again: the mother impregnated and deprived of another calf, and another, and another, while the calf grows to maturity and becomes a mother herself (cows can give birth from two to three years old). The mother's milk production capacity, having been pushed to its limits (up to ten times what she would have produced naturally), declines at around five or six years old, and at that point she will be sent for slaughter. She could have lived to be 15 or 20.

Increasingly, dairy cows are being subjected to 'zero-grazing': permanently housed inside and never allowed out to graze. This can lead to mastitis (infection of the udders) and lameness, both of which are extremely painful.

And, just as male chicks are deemed essentially worthless, so too are male calves: 90,000 are shot at birth every year in the UK; others are kept alive for between four and five months to produce veal (and fed an iron-deficient diet in order to keep them borderline anaemic and ensure that the veal is the pale colour consumers like and expect).

Beef cattle fare a little better, in the same way that layer chickens fare better than broiler ones. They are mainly allowed out to graze in the open in the UK (though in many parts of Europe they are kept inside far more often and fattened on a high grain diet), but when they reach the required weight they are slaughtered. This usually takes place at around 18 months old – again, well short of their natural lifespan.

And the methods of slaughter are just as flawed as they are with poultry. The cows are supposed to be stunned with a shot from a bolt gun before being shackled, hoisted and having their throats cut. But the stunning often fails, meaning that cows have to undergo either multiple shots from the bolt gun and/or exsanguination while still conscious.

PIGS

Despite their popular image as dirty and slow-witted, the bluffer should know that pigs are naturally both clean and intelligent: studies have shown them to be smarter than dogs and capable of solving problems as well as chimpanzees do. (The phrase 'their popular image as dirty and slow-witted' obviously refers to the pigs rather than to bluffers, who as any fule kno have excellent standards of both personal hygiene and mental agility.) They are sociable and gregarious, and like to maintain physical contact with other pigs when sleeping. (Still on the pigs here, obviously.) But three-quarters of pigs in the UK are factory farmed,[12] and conditions are no better for them than they are for chickens or cows.

Just as chickens are debeaked to prevent them from harming each other, piglets have their tails docked and their teeth clipped or ground down – even though pigs in the wild rarely harm each other, and do so in captivity as a direct response to the overcrowding and lack of stimuli.

And just as mother cows are separated from their calves, so too with mother pigs and their calves. Pigs are forced to give birth in farrowing crates (illegal in several European countries, but still standard practice in the UK), which allows piglets to suckle her but does

12 Compassion in World Farming.

not permit her to nuzzle them as the bars get in the way. The piglets are taken from her after 28 days; that is, a third or a quarter of the time she would spend weaning them naturally. As with cows, the separation causes both parties distress, with mother and child repeatedly and loudly calling for each other.

Like chickens and cows, pigs could live to be around 20; like chickens and cows, they are killed a long way short of this. Mothers typically undergo between three and five pregnancies before being slaughtered at around 18 months to two years old; piglets are often killed between four and six months.[13]

And, as with chickens and cows, the slaughtering process is flawed and often painful. Pigs in particular are liable to become distressed in such situations, and many slaughterhouse workers have stories of pigs who've tried to jump out of their enclosures, smashed themselves against walls, tried to chew through gates or lift them off their hinges with their snouts, and so on.

Few schoolkids have ever said to their careers officer: 'I really, really want to work in an abattoir.' Working conditions are often atrocious and the strain is intense. …

---

13 Kate Schuler, *Veganuary: How to Go Vegan*, 2017.

At this point, it may be worth remembering that slaughterhouse workers don't exactly have it easy themselves. They, having established his or her classical credentials earlier (Ovid, Plutarch, Pythagoras etc.), can point out that in ancient Greece slaughtering animals was the job of priests; in the modern industrialised world, it's entrusted to minimum wage workers (often immigrants, illegal or otherwise, who are less likely to kick up a fuss, join unions or bring legal action). Few schoolkids have ever said to their careers officer: 'I really, really want to work in an abattoir.' Working conditions are often atrocious and the strain is intense, both physically (machine-related injuries and carpal tunnel syndrome) and psychologically (post-traumatic stress disorder and emotional numbing). In many slaughterhouses, annual staff turnover runs at more than 100%. This is a brutal job all round.

FISH

Ah, the non-bluffer will say, but fishing's different, isn't it? Not really, the bluffer can reply, and if you think it is, that's probably because of your schema which sees cold-blooded fish as somehow less worthy than warm-blooded mammals. Both open sea and farmed fishing take place under conditions which are cruel to the fish. As vegan author Kate Schuler writes: 'Commercial fishing vessels can capture tens of thousands of fish at a time, with animals becoming exhausted as they desperately try to outswim the net. When pulled to the surface, those at the bottom are crushed by the weight of fish above them. The rapid change in pressure causes their swim bladders to overinflate, and their stomachs and intestines to be pushed out through their mouths and anuses. Their eyes distort, bulge and can be pushed out of their sockets. The animals are then dropped onto the ship's deck, where those who are still alive will suffocate – a process that can take several minutes.'[14]

Fish farms are no better. 'In fish farms, fish are packed into small, often filthy enclosures. The overcrowded conditions cause a third of them to die, and an array of chemicals is used to try to prevent even more from succumbing. In this stressful environment, many fish will bite off the fins, tails and eyes of others, a distressing and destructive behaviour seen in other factory-farmed animals. Despite an ever-increasing number of studies that show aquatic species can feel pain, there are still no welfare laws governing the humane slaughter of fish at sea, and in most countries there are no welfare requirements for slaughter on farms, either. With little or no legal protection, some truly terrible things are done to aquatic species. Lobsters and crabs may be boiled alive, while farmed shrimps are deliberately blinded in a procedure designed to boost their fertility. "Eyestalk ablation" happens in almost every shrimp production facility in the world.'[15]

There is also a substantial amount of collateral damage, or 'bycatch', in net fishing – that is, species not seen as commercially valuable but caught anyway. The global fishing industry accounts for around 20m tonnes of bycatch each year, including an estimated 300,000

14 Schuler, ibid.
15 Schuler, ibid. The removal of shrimps' eyestalks triggers the maturing of their ovaries.

whales, dolphins and porpoises: all caught and killed before they can be returned to the water.[16] The bluffer can use the word 'bycatch' liberally when discussing fishing, though must make sure not to confuse it with some typically butterfingered fielding from English cricketers.

THE COUNTER-ARGUMENTS

The bluffer should always be keen to deploy the phrase 'on the other hand', usually accompanied by a thoughtful stroke of the chin and/or expression of infinite sagacity, and this is an ideal opportunity for such scales-balancing/bigger-picture-seeing.

There are several arguments in defence of factory farming:

- they generate revenue and employment, both directly (people working on the farms) and indirectly (those working in ancillary sectors such as deliveries);
- they take up less space, certainly *pro rata*, than traditional farms;
- and they allow for the most efficient rearing, feeding and slaughter of animals, which in turn helps to keep the price of the finished product affordable for those on lower incomes.

These are all cogent arguments. As far as veganism is concerned, however, none of them begins to address the animal welfare concerns.

16 Schuler, ibid.

'I'm healthier and happier than I've ever been. Wish I did it [gone vegan] sooner.'

Lewis Hamilton, May 2019

COUCH POTATO (REASONS TO BE VEGAN, PART 2)

HEALTH

It may sound counter-intuitive that being vegan (and therefore cutting out a large range of possible nutrition) is good for your health, but there is plenty of evidence that this is the case. (The bluffer should, of course, love anything that sounds counter-intuitive, for it gives them the opportunity to show that what appears counter-intuitive is actually counter-counter-intuitive: or, to cut a long word short, intuitive.)

The World Health Organisation states that the first step to healthy eating is to 'eat a nutritious diet based on a variety of foods originating mainly from plants rather than animals', and in 2015 ranked processed meat as a Group

1 carcinogen ('there is enough evidence to conclude that it can cause cancer in humans' – the same category as cigarettes, alcohol and asbestos) and red meat as a Group 2A carcinogen ('there is strong evidence that it can cause cancer in humans, but at present it is not conclusive' – the same category as malaria, bitumen and creosote). This is all rather alarming for carnivores, to say the least.

A 2016 study suggested that a global move to a vegan diet (still strictly hypothetical, of course: *see Romaines to be Seen*) would avert 8.1 million premature deaths per year.[17] That's the equivalent of the population of London. One of the world's great cities, wiped out. Every year.

But that's enough about death-by-diet. Veganism can help in the following areas:

- **Diabetes.** A 2019 Harvard study concluded that a vegan diet can cut the risk of developing type 2 diabetes by almost a quarter.
- **Prostate cancer.** Vegan diets have been linked to a 35% lower risk of prostate cancer.[18] At present, according to the shock statistic underlying the advertising campaign launched by prostatecanceruk.org, one man dies every 45 minutes from prostate cancer in the UK, and 1 in 8 men will be diagnosed with prostate cancer in their lifetime. And something as natural as a plant-based diet could save their lives. …
- **Heart disease and stroke** are less common among vegans, who eat less cholesterol and saturated fat

17 Oxford Martin Programme on the Future of Food.
18 World Cancer Research Fund study, reported in *The Independent*, March 2016.

than omnivores (there's no cholesterol in plants) and exhibit fewer instances of high blood pressure.[19]

- *Obesity.* Vegans on average have lower body mass indices.[20]
- *General health.* Participants in Veganuary often report that even a month eating vegan food improves their digestion, energy, hair, mental clarity, sinuses, skin and sleep.[21]

Most government bodies in the developed world (including the five main English-speaking nations: Australia, Canada, New Zealand, the UK and the US) endorse well-planned vegan diets as appropriate for everyone, including infants and pregnant women. The German Society for Nutrition, however, does not recommend vegan diets for children or adolescents, or during pregnancy and breastfeeding. (*The Bluffer's Guide* is striving with every sinew it possesses not to make a cheap joke about what else one could expect from a nation whose idea of fine dining is bratwurst and pig's knuckle.)

The two salient points here ('salient points' being another mainstay of the bluffer's general approach to life) are 'well-planned' and 'the developed world'. Vegan food is not in and of itself a perfect source of nutrition, and

19 Study carried out by the Mayo Clinic in Rochester, Minnesota, reported in the *Journal of the American College of Cardiology*, 2019.

20 2016 *Journal of General Internal Medicine* meta-analysis of randomised trials on the effect of vegetarian diets on obesity rates. Vegetarian diets achieved significantly greater weight loss than energy restriction diets, and subgroup analysis found that vegan diets produced greater weight loss than vegetarian diets.

21 Schuler, ibid.

unbalanced and/or overly processed vegan diets can be as damaging as their non-vegan counterparts. The chapter *Salad Gold* takes a closer look at this issue. Moreover, vegan diets may not be appropriate in developing countries where people have much less access to widespread sources of plant-based nutrition, and therefore where meat, eggs and dairy may be not so much damaging luxuries as vital sources of food, enabling children in particular to develop physically and mentally in a way they would otherwise have been denied.

The two salient points here ('salient points' being another mainstay of the bluffer's general approach to life) are 'well-planned' and 'the developed world'.

Even (or perhaps especially) sportsmen and women can benefit from a vegan diet. Lewis Hamilton may be one of the most famous vegan sportspeople, but he is by no means the only one. Other vegan sportspeople include: the tennis players Serena and Venus Williams; the footballers (soccer players, if you're an American reading this) Jermain Defoe, Fabian Delph and Jack Wilshere; the American footballer (football player, if you're an American (still) reading this) Colin Kaepernick; the skater Meagan Duhamel; Dana Glowacka, who holds the women's world record for maintaining the plank position (4 hours 20 minutes! Most people, even relatively fit ones, couldn't manage 4 minutes 20 seconds); and ultramarathon champions Scott Jurek and Rich Roll (both of whom credit much of their success to their vegan diets).

Nor is it simply individual personal health which veganism can improve. Global health is also at play here, particularly the risk of pandemics due to increasing human resistance to antibiotics. A 2015 report stated that 'the precise quantity of antimicrobials [a wider category of agent of which antibiotics are an example: the kind of distinction which, when judiciously deployed, suggests measureless depths to the bluffer's knowledge – and indeed those depths may well be measureless, just not quite in the way the bluffer would like others to think] used in food production globally is difficult to estimate, but the evidence suggests that it is at least as great as the amount used by humans. Indeed in some parts of the world antimicrobial use is far greater in animals than in humans; in the US, for instance, more than 70 percent of medically important antibiotics are used in animals.

'The risks associated with the high use of antimicrobials are threefold. Firstly, it presents the risk that drug-resistant strains are passed on through direct contact between humans and animals (notably farmers). Secondly, these drug-resistant strains have the potential to be passed onto humans more generally through the food chain, i.e. when consumers prepare or eat the meat itself. Finally, there is a further indirect threat to human health as result of animal excretion.

Both resistant bacteria, as well as significant volumes of antibiotics consumed, are then excreted by animals (with most of the active ingredient unmetabolised). This both releases resistant bacteria into the environment as well as causing the environment to be tainted with antibiotics, providing further opportunities for exposure to bacteria and creating additional selective pressure that leads to the development of drug resistance.'[22]

As Foer says, 'there is scientific consensus that new viruses, which move between farmed animals and humans, will be a major global health threat into the foreseeable future. The concern is not only bird flu or swine flu or whatever-comes-next, but the entire class of 'zoonotic' (animal-to-human or vice versa) pathogens – especially viruses that move between humans, chickens, turkeys, and pigs.'[23]

We have already seen how diseases can spread from animals to humans: the H1N1 swine flu pandemic of 2009–10 (itself, as the bluffer will know, a descendant of the Spanish flu pandemic which killed between 50m and 100m people in the aftermath of the First World War), and the H5N1 avian flu strain which is primarily but not totally confined to Asia. The more that humans consume antibiotics in farmed meat, the more vulnerable they become to mutating antibiotic-resistant strains of animal flu. Plants do not carry antibiotics the same way animals do. No one is ever going to die from broccoli flu or spinach flu, and tofu will never become to-flu.

22 'Antimicrobials in agriculture and the environment: reducing unnecessary use and waste.' *Review on Antimicrobial Resistance*, December 2015.
23 Foer, ibid.

ROCKET SCIENCE (REASONS TO BE VEGAN, PART 3)

Going vegan helps the environment: it's as simple as that. The extent to which it helps the environment is a matter of debate (when is it not, with scientists?), but that there is an overall beneficial effect is beyond doubt. 'Avoiding meat and dairy,' said a 2018 Oxford University study, 'is the single biggest way to reduce your impact on Earth.' A Greenpeace report from the same year concluded that 'global meat and dairy production and consumption must be cut in half by 2050 to avoid dangerous climate change and keep the Paris Agreement on track. If left unchecked, agriculture is projected to produce 52% of global greenhouse gas emissions in the coming decades, 70% of which will come from meat and dairy.' And, according to one study, if every family in the

UK removed meat from just one meal a week, it would have the same environmental impact as taking 16m cars off the road.[24]

Livestock is, directly and indirectly, one of the major contributors to emissions, and the bluffer should know about both. Directly, because fermentation by ruminants (cows, sheep, goats etc.) produces methane (CH_4), a greenhouse gas (GHG) which accounts for only 14.5% of anthropogenic (human-caused) GHG emissions[25] but which has a global warming potential 28 times that of carbon dioxide (CO_2).[26]

And indirectly, because so many resources go into raising farm animals rather than humans. We could feed twice as many humans if we did not feed farmed animals but rather consumed the yield ourselves.[27] The resources being used include:

- *Energy.* The average UK meat-eater's diet accounts for almost twice as much CO_2 (2,055kg p/a) as the average UK vegan's (1,055kg p/a) and is appreciably higher than the average vegetarian's (1,391kg).[28]
- *Food.* 'Animals are inefficient converters of feed to meat. In simple terms, we get back less than we put in. Pigs, for example, require 8.4kg of feed to produce

24 The Meatless Farm Co., May 2019.
25 Food and Agriculture Organisation of the United Nations, 2019.
26 Institute of Biology, Environmental and Rural Sciences, Aberystwyth University, February 2019.
27 A.T. Kearney, 2019.
28 European Prospective Investigation into Cancer and Nutrition (EPIC) – Oxford study, 2014.

1kg of meat, while chickens require 3.4kg of feed to produce 1kg. For every 100 calories of grain we feed to farmed animals, we get back only about 40 new calories of milk, 22 calories of eggs, 12 of chicken, 10 of pork or 3 of beef.'[29] 'It takes 2,000lb [900kg] of grain to produce enough meat and other livestock products to feed a person for a year. However, if that person ate the grain directly, rather than via animal products, it would take only 400lb (180kg) of grain.'[30] Some 93% of the world's soya goes to feeding animals rather than humans. Nor is it just plants that animals consume: they also account for around 70% of the global fish catch,[31] which itself is a major contributor to the erosion of natural maritime habitats and damage to oceanic ecosystems.

- **Water.** Though avocados have the highest water footprint of all fruits and vegetables at 1,981m³/ton, this is still much less than those of eggs (3,300m³/ton), chicken meat (4,300m³/ton), pork and bacon (6,000m³/ton), and beef (15,400m³/ton).[32]

- **Land.** The veteran campaigner George Monbiot quotes Harvard research when he says 'an astonishing 55% of UK cropping land (land that is ploughed and seeded) is used to grow feed for livestock, rather than food for humans. If our grazing land was allowed to revert to natural ecosystems, and the land currently used to grow feed for livestock was used for grains,

29 Schuler, ibid.
30 Joy, ibid.
31 Joy, ibid.
32 *The Ecologist*, May 2019.

beans, fruit, nuts and vegetables for humans, this switch would allow the UK to absorb an astonishing quantity of carbon. This would be equivalent, altogether, the paper estimates, to absorbing nine years of our total current emissions. And farming in this country could then feed everyone, without the need for imports. A plant-based diet would make the difference between the UK's current failure to meet its international commitments, and success.'[33] 'Whether human beings survive this century and the next, whether other life forms can live alongside us: more than anything, this depends on the way we eat. We can cut our consumption of everything else almost to zero and still we will drive living systems to collapse unless we change our diet.'[34]

The disagreement among scientists and campaigners as to the environmental benefits of going vegan tend to focus on the numbers rather than the proposition itself. Bjorn Lomborg, former director of Denmark's Environmental Assessment Institute, says that 'a non-meat diet will reduce an individual's emissions by 540kg of carbon dioxide. For the average person in the industrialised world, that means cutting emissions by just 4.3%. But even this still overstates the effect because it ignores an age-old economic phenomenon known as the rebound effect. Vegetarian diets are slightly cheaper, and the saved money will likely be spent on other goods

33 *The Guardian*, August 2019.
34 *The Guardian*, 2018.

and services that cause additional greenhouse-gas emissions. In the US, vegetarians save about 7% and in the UK about 15% of their food budgets. A Swedish study showed a vegetarian diet is 10% cheaper, freeing up about 2% of an individual's total budget.

'That extra spending will cause more carbon-dioxide emissions and cancel out half the saved emissions from going vegetarian, the study concludes. Instead of going completely vegetarian for the rest of your life, you could reduce greenhouse-gas emissions by the exact same amount using the EU Emissions Trading System (always a useful reference for the bluffer, not least because so few people actually know what it is or does) while eating anything you want. There are many good reasons to eat less meat. But making a huge difference to the climate isn't one of them.'[35] (Of course, Lomborg – himself a vegetarian for ethical reasons – was discussing vegetarian rather than vegan diets, but in terms of environmental costs there is far less difference between vegetarian and vegan than there is between vegetarian and meat.)

The environmental writer Matt Ridley points out that 'much of the plant material we grow on arable land cannot be eaten by human beings – straw, for example. Plus cows, pigs and chickens turn the indigestible stuff into manure without which soil conservation would be harder and organic farming all but impossible. Professor Imke de Boer of Wageningen University, in the Netherlands, argues that the most carbon-efficient

35 *New Europe*, November 2018.

agriculture must include some animals. Much of this planet cannot be used for growing crops, but can produce fodder for sheep, cattle, goats, camels and chickens.

'The hills of Scotland, Wales and the Lake District, for example, are not suitable for wheat, nor is much of the Middle East and Central Asia. Without these animals, we would not only ruin many farming communities, but have to plough and plant a lot more land elsewhere to grow the protein and fats that we otherwise get from animals – and that would mean destroying more forests and wetlands, because unlike sheep and cows, those crops need well-watered, fertile soil. Bad idea!'[36] (If you can read those last two words in any voice other than Donald Trump's, you're a better person than this particular writer.)

And Rob Greenfield, creator of the Food Waste Fiasco campaign 'that strives to end food waste and hunger in the US', points out that 'all plant-based diets are not created equal. A person who lives off the land and includes meat in their diet can have a smaller environmental impact than a person who lives in the city and eats all plant-based food (most of which may be packaged and shipped in). Plant-based diets often include food that is shipped from halfway around the world burning fossil fuels, food that is covered in packaging which is very resource-intensive (whether it's recycled or not), and food that contains harmful ingredients like palm oil.

'[For example] Louisiana is a state with many self-

36 *Daily Telegraph*, August 2018.

sufficient people. For many of them, the bayou is their bloodline and they live off this land. Their diets include alligators, crayfish, fish, rabbit, deer and so much more. These swamps are absolutely teeming with life and I believe that when they hunt it responsibly, these folk can eat a more Earth-friendly diet than a person living in the city eating a plant-based diet from the supermarket. And a more environmentally responsible diet than going to the stores they have available in the area, where there really isn't access to quality plant-based foods.'[37]

(For the bluffer to quote a Danish academic, a British journalist and an American campaigner, should suggest that there's plenty more where that came from: that there's a great, almost limitless, breadth and depth to his or her knowledge, that like an iceberg only a small part of that knowledge is visible at any one time, and that the bluffer in every way Sees the Bigger Picture. That's our hope, anyway.)

37 www.robgreenfield.tv, July 2015.

'Vegan food is soul food in its truest form. Soul food means to feed the soul. And to me, your soul is your intent. If your intent is pure, you are pure.'

Erykah Badu, American singer-songwriter

SALAD GOLD: THE VEGAN DIET

With one exception (see below), a vegan diet can provide every nutrient and vitamin essential to a healthy lifestyle. A vegan who's eating badly is not doing so because they're vegan: they're doing so because they haven't balanced their diet properly.

When it comes to food, vegans are asked two questions above all, and the bluffer should know what these are and how to answer them. In a world of political correctness, veganism has its own PC: that is, protein and calcium. Since protein is associated with meat and calcium with dairy, non-vegans tend to assume the vegan is not just lacking these two vital nutrients but hankering after them like a thirst-crazed man marooned in the desert seeking water or stalking supermarket aisles like a plant-based zombie.

HOW DO YOU GET ENOUGH PROTEIN?

Easily. It's just that where omnivores receive only half their daily protein from plant-based foods, and vegetarians two-thirds of theirs, vegans by definition receive 100% of their protein this way. There's protein in legumes (soy beans and everything which is made from them (such as tofu), black beans, lentils and chickpeas), grains (quinoa, rice, corn, barley and wheat), nuts (Brazil nuts, walnuts, almonds, cashews, peanuts, pistachios) and seeds. Soy beans and quinoa in particular are excellent sources of protein; in fact, they're called 'complete proteins' because they contain all essential amino acids in amounts that meet or exceed human requirements. 'Plant proteins are much better for us than animal proteins, as plants are packed with nutrients but include none of the cholesterol.'[38]

For some reason, the slightest mention – even, perhaps, the very concept – of quinoa enrages some non-vegans. Perhaps it's the overtones of smug North London progressives. Perhaps it's the fact that they can't pronounce it properly. Perhaps it's both. Either way, it does wind people up. Whether or not you choose to use this or avoid it depends on how much you like winding these particular people up.

HOW DO YOU GET ENOUGH CALCIUM?

Again, easily. There's calcium in kale, watercress, broccoli, cabbage, okra, sweet potato, sesame seeds and

38 *Vegan Life: Cruelty-Free Food, Fashion, Beauty and Home.* Jo Peters, 2019.

tahini, pulses, bread (calcium is added to white and brown flour by law), dried fruit, and dairy replacements such as fortified plant milks and soy yoghurt. Calcium-set tofu is also a good source. Many animal products contain calcium mainly because the animals have ingested it from plants, so the bluffer can make airy pronouncements about cutting out the middleman (middlemanimal?) here. If elephants can maintain healthy bones on a plant-based diet, so too can humans.

OTHER DIETARY ASPECTS OF VEGANISM

Iron

Iron (essential for the production of red blood cells) is absorbed more easily into the body from meat than it is from plants, but there are still plenty of good vegan iron sources: pulses; soybean tempeh (not to be confused with rapper Tinie Tempah), black beans, lentils and chickpeas; wholemeal bread and flour; nuts; oatmeal; dried fruit; iron-fortified breakfast cereals; and dark green leafy vegetables such as watercress, broccoli and spinach.

(In fact, the bluffer can afford to go off-piste a little here and opine that *Popeye* can be seen very much as early pro-vegan propaganda. The title character gets all his strength from spinach. His girlfriend is called Olive Oyl and his child ward Swee'Pea. And Bluto, his antagonist, is clearly a meat-eater, and yet always finds himself coming off second best to PPP – Plant-Powered Popeye.)

Iron is absorbed more easily when consumed alongside Vitamin C, so wash down your meal with a glass of orange juice (champagne or vodka optional).

Omega-3 and -6 fatty acids

These are two polyunsaturated fats which help reduce the risk of heart disease and are most often found in fish oil. Vegan sources of omega-3 fatty acids include oils (flaxseed, rapeseed, soya), chia seeds and walnuts. Omega-6 can also be found in sunflower oil.

Vitamin B12

Needed for the formation and maturation of red blood cells, the synthesis of DNA, and maintaining a healthy nervous system function, Vitamin B12 is found naturally only in foods from animal sources, and is therefore the one nutrient which cannot be found in raw plant-based foods. As such, vegans need to ingest it either through fortified food (yeast extract spreads such as Marmite, fortified cereals/plant milks) or vitamin supplements.

RECIPES

If you want vegan recipes, there are plenty available online, not to mention a whole raft of vegan cookbooks available from all good bookshops, some terrible bookshops too, and of course from online behemoths which may or may not be named after South American rivers and may or may not minimise their global tax burden in strict accordance with the laws of the countries in which they operate. But you won't find any recipes here. Do I look like Jamie Oliver? (Don't answer that.)

A common complaint among non-vegans is that vegan food is bland and rather 'meh'. There are two obvious ways in which the bluffer can respond here.

Firstly, lots of non-vegan food is pretty bland too. Secondly, the way for vegan food to become more delicious is for more people to turn vegan, thus obliging vegan food manufacturers/restaurants/cafes to up their game or risk being frozen out by the competition. In this respect it is rather, if the phrase is not too inappropriate (and the bluffer may allow themself a small satisfied chuckle at the woeful pun about to be unleashed here), a chicken and egg situation.

THE ACCIDENTAL VEGAN

Bluffers can also point out the logical conundrum that vegan food doesn't have to be branded as such, or specifically vegan. There are plenty of 'accidentally vegan' foodstuffs out there which feature heavily in many people's everyday diets and just happen not to contain any meat, fish, dairy, eggs or honey. With the usual caveats that the manufacturers may change the ingredients at any time and you should always check the label, the following are vegan even if you don't instinctively think of them as such:

- most bread (look out for eggs and milk)
- most pasta (ditto re eggs and milk)
- most crisps (except cheesy flavours and some meaty ones too)
- most cereals (though look out for Vitamin D3, gelatine and milk powder)
- most peanut butter
- most instant noodles

- most stir-fry sauces (some contain anchovies)
- most spices
- most spirits (so if all else fails the bluffer can simply drink himself insensible before grabbing the nearest person in a headlock and informing them that 'You're my best mate. You are, you know. I love you.')
- most crackers (check for cheese)
- most Quorn (though some contains eggs)
- some sweets, including Starbursts (the old school bluffer will still insist on referring to these as 'Opal Fruits', naturally, rebranding be damned), Millions, Jelly Tots, Flying Saucers, Sherbet Fountains, Skittles, Turkish Delight and Haribo Sour Rainbow Strips/Twists
- some chocolate, including Cadbury Bournville Plain Chocolate, many Green & Blacks varieties (Dark Chocolate, Hazelnut & Currant, Ginger, Maya Gold, Espresso, Spiced Chilli, Lemon, Mint), Lindt Excellence – 70%, 85% and 90% Dark Chocolate, Fry's Chocolate Cream and Tesco Dark Chocolate Mint Thins. Sadly Ferrero Rocher contains milk, so although the ambassador may indeed be spoiling us, he's not a vegan.
- some biscuits, including Hobnobs, Ginger Nuts, Fox's Party Rings and Bourbons.
- some cakes, including Lidl's Bramley apple pies and Mr Kipling Treacle Tart, Jam Tarts, Apple and Blackcurrant Pies
- and even some fast food (McDonalds and Burger King fries, Subway's veggie delight, and Pizza Hut, Dominos and Pizza Express all do takeaway pizza with vegan cheese.

For vegans, of course, what to avoid in foodstuffs is as important as what to include. It's not merely the obvious (that large hunk of gammon is a bit of a giveaway), but the smaller ingredients which may not be obvious until and unless you read the label. Non-vegan ingredients include:

- aspic (from animal products and gelatine)
- carmine (crushed beetles)
- casein (milk)
- castoreum (beavers' scent glands)
- cod liver oil (fish (you don't say))
- collagen (skin, ligaments and bones of cattle, fish, poultry and swine)
- elastin (cattle ligaments and blood vessels)
- isinglass (fish bladders)
- keratin (skin, ligaments and bones of cattle, fish, poultry and swine)
- pepsin (pigs' stomachs)
- rennet (stomachs of newly born calves)
- shellac (insect secretion)
- suet (cattle and sheep kidneys)
- tallow (animal fat).

'We do not need to eat animals, wear animals, or use animals for entertainment purposes, and our only defence of these uses is our pleasure, amusement, and convenience.'

Gary Francione, animal rights legal scholar

KALE OF DUTY: THE VEGAN LIFESTYLE

As mentioned in *Cool Beans*, the bluffer should emphasise that veganism is not merely a matter of diet, of what to and what not to eat. It's a wider, more overarching philosophy than that, best summed up in the Vegan Society's own definition of veganism as a 'way of living which seeks to exclude – as far as is possible and practicable – all forms of exploitation of, and cruelty to, animals for food, clothing or any other purpose; and by extension, promotes the development and use of animal-free alternatives for the benefit of humans, animals and the environment'.

Vegans therefore take care to avoid animal exploitation in the following areas:

Clothes

Many typical clothing materials are anathema for vegans, including feathers (often plucked from the birds rather than collected once moulted), fur, leather, silk, snakeskin, suede, wool (and variations such as cashmere, angora and mohair). Vegans prefer to wear clothes made from non-animal-derived materials such as canvas, cotton, denim, hemp, linen, pleather (artificial leather), polyester, rubber (settle down at the back there), ground seaweed fibre and vinyl. Even if shoes are made from non-animal products, any glue used in their manufacture might have animal ingredients.

The days of vegan clothing being lumpen shapeless afterthoughts are long gone. Many designers, including Gucci, Stella McCartney and Donatella Versace, are using vegan alternatives in their clothes; and many high street retailers are also becoming increasingly vegan-friendly. Dr Martens vegan boots, which replace the leather uppers with synthetic polyurethane plastic, now account for 4% of the company's sales, and CEO Kenny Wilson says that their popularity has increased by 'multiple hundreds of percent' in recent years.[39] And, as everyone old enough to remember Alexei Sayle on *The Young Ones* will know, 'It's not class or ideology/colour, creed or roots/The only thing that unites us/Is Dr Martens boots.' (If the bluffer is not old enough, he should nonetheless make it appear as though he's au fait with all 1980s alternative comedy programmes.)

---

39 *The Guardian*, August 2019.

The days of vegan clothing being lumpen shapeless afterthoughts are long gone. Many designers, including Gucci, Stella McCartney and Donatella Versace, are using vegan alternatives in their clothes; and many high street retailers are also becoming increasingly vegan-friendly.

Personal care items

Since soap is usually made from tallow (animal fat), vegans use specifically vegan soap made from olive oil. Shampoo, moisturiser, shaving foam and toothpaste often contain collagen, making them unsuitable for vegans. Carmine is used to make red and pink shades in many cosmetics, so this must be avoided too.

If an item carries either the Vegan Society's sunflower logo and/or the PETA bunny, it's certified as vegan and free from animal testing. The Vegan Society's criteria for vegan certification are that the product contains no animal products, and that neither the finished item nor its ingredients have been tested on animals by, or on behalf of, the manufacturer or by anyone over whom the manufacturer has control. The society's website contains a list of certified products. (If an item has a leaping bunny, it has not been tested on animals but may not be vegan.)

Circuses and zoos

Fewer circuses use animals these days, but there are still some (and more so abroad than in the UK). Zoos – at least well-run ones – do have some educational and conservational merit (this itself may be a profitable tangent for bluffer discussion), and the workers are in general committed to the welfare of their charges, but all animals in zoos are by definition confined in conditions totally alien to their natural environment, and their behaviour often suffers because of this.

Animal transport

Horse-drawn carriage rides in cities are rarely, if ever, paragons of animal welfare standards. The horses are often kept in suboptimal conditions: the noise of traffic and people causes them stress, the fumes from urban emissions harm their respiratory systems, and repeated trotting on unyielding tarmac risks injuring their legs (horses are usually worked on softer ground). Donkeys in seaside resorts generally have an even worse time of it.

Blood sports

Goes without saying, really. Fox hunting, game shooting, fishing, bullfighting … all these are total anathema to vegans.

Going on holiday

It can be hard to know what products are vegan-friendly in foreign countries, where labelling is different and the language may be unfamiliar. The chapter *I Herb It*

Through the Grapevine gives an overview of vegan-friendly cities round the world – cities, with their younger and more progressive populations, unsurprisingly tend to be more vegan-friendly than rural areas – and Google Translate will give you the words for vegan staples in pretty much any language you choose (including Latin, which will be useful if you're ever holidaying with Jacob Rees-Mogg). Since vegan food may be hard to find in transport termini and on planes/trains/buses, it may be wise to take your own while en route just in case.

'I quickly learned that going vegan required compassion for myself as much as for the animals and I urge you to be gentle with yourself as you work towards integrating veganism seamlessly into your life.'

Kate Schuler

TURNING OVER A NEW LEAF

So, the bluffer might frequently be asked, how best do you become vegan? As so often in bluffing, the answer should subtly hint at a judicious but concise weighing of the various options, a recognition that there are several different possible avenues and the best one depends very much on the identity and character of the person taking it. 'Go at your own pace', 'horses for courses' and similar phrases should be dropped in at opportune intervals. All this, of course, should be prefaced with the old bluffer's standby: 'Well, X, I'm glad you asked me that question …' (This is also, of course, a well-worn politician's phrase, not least because all politicians are bluffers, but that should not taint what is essentially a noble calling.)

The first thing to do when considering making the switch is to be as informed as possible and learn as much as you can – for example, by reading this book.

Forewarned is forearmed, time spent in reconnaissance is seldom wasted, prior planning prevents piss-poor performance; anyone who's ever had an uncle in the army will know these all too well.

There's a wealth of information out there – books, documentaries, social media, blogs, forums – all of which you can use to help you decide whether and when you want to make the leap. Be sure not just that you want to do it but why you want to do it; if personal health is your main motivator, for example, it may be easier to give up (if you don't feel the health benefits quickly enough) than it would be if you were driven by animal welfare.

Decision taken, there are three main options: the slow replacement, the halfway house, and the full-on leap.

THE SLOW REPLACEMENT

You slowly and gradually cut out animal products from your diet. Begin with the easiest ones – i.e. those you'll miss the least – and leave your favourites till the end. For every animal product you ditch, replace it with a plant-based one. The animal/non-animal balance in your diet will slowly tip in favour of the latter.

- *Pros*: easing your way into a major diet change reduces the physiological and psychological shock to your system.
- *Cons:* it's easy to get stuck near the end when you don't want to give up your favourite non-vegan food and are tempted to think: 'Ah well, I'm 90% of the way there

and that's better than nothing, it doesn't matter if I have a cheeseburger/minute steak/full Sunday roast with all the trimmings from time to time.'

THE HALFWAY HOUSE

You go vegetarian first, and then vegan after a while, either by cutting out dairy and eggs in one go or one food group at a time. Remove all meat from your diet, remembering to fill the gap with increased plant-based foods rather than bulking up ovo-lacto consumption.

- *Pros:* as with the Slow Replacement, it's both physiologically and psychologically easier to do it in stages.
- *Cons:* you may find yourself marooned on Vegetarian Island and unwilling to make the final leap. It's better than nothing, of course, but less than what you intended.

THE FULL-ON LEAP

Just as it says on the (vegan) tin: a brutal, immediate transition. Omnivore one day and vegan the next. Slash and burn, scorched earth, cold tofurkey. Use direct vegan alternatives to animal-based foods – vegan burgers, vegan cheeses etc. – if need be to soothe at least some of the shock.

- *Pros:* the prospect of backsliding or stalling is minimised.

- *Cons:* without proper planning you risk an unbalanced diet, which in turn will make you feel that maybe this vegan lark isn't all it's cracked up to be, which in turn may tempt you to give up as fully and immediately as you started and go back to being an omnivore.

You will need to eat more than you're used to: vegan foods tend to be lower in calories than animal-based ones. You may be more flatulent (in which case, blame it on the dog. Remember to check that you have a dog before trying this).

The bluffer will, of course, know the similarities between the various routes as well as the differences. Whichever route you choose, your body will need time to adapt and you may notice certain physical changes. For a start, you will need to eat more than you're used to: vegan foods tend to be lower in calories than animal-based ones. You may be more flatulent (in which case, blame it on the dog. Remember to check that you have a dog before trying this). Your bowel movements may be more frequent and/or looser, due to the higher fibre content of a vegan diet. You may have more energy (courtesy of removing processed meat from your diet), but you may also feel more tired (getting your diet right and ensuring you have enough nutrition).

Since veganism is about lifestyle as much as it is about diet, you will also need to make changes to your wider life too. Personal care products, like food, are easily replaceable and have a relatively short shelf life, but clothes are a different matter. Do you throw out all your non-vegan clothes and fully veganise your wardrobe in one go? Can you afford to? Or do you keep using what you already have, recognising both that in vegan terms the damage has already long been done and that buying anything new has an environmental as well as a financial cost, and replace items when they wear out as you would do normally?

Unless you're a hermit (which, let's face it, is pretty tempting sometimes) you'll have to deal with the reactions of friends, family, colleagues, and some bloke on Twitter who just wants a pop, nothing personal, just bantz, Jeez, lighten up, some people really can't take a joke. Some will be hostile, some sneering, some dismissive, some interested, and some just looking to take the piss. In general, it's best to stand your ground, not rise to provocations, and laugh along with any jokes which come free from malice. Don't proselytise, don't accuse, and don't be afraid to change the subject if you've had enough.

Also, don't be surprised if somewhere down the line someone who's hitherto shown no interest in veganism comes to talk to you about it after being impressed/ intrigued/inspired by your example. You're very unlikely to convert anyone on the spot – remember the schema from *Peas of Mind* – but you may plant a seed (pun intended) in someone's head and prompt them to think differently.

'Remember also that every time you pick a vegan option when you're out and about, you are influencing the people around you. Depending on your current diet, you could save between 100 and 200 animals every year by going vegan.'

When going out to eat, more and more restaurants have vegan options on their menus. Some even have separate vegan menus, though they may not produce them unless you ask. If there really are no vegan options, ask the waiter what the chef can prepare which is suitable. When at a big family meal (such as Christmas) offer to cook a vegan dish, not just so you'll have something to eat but also to show non-vegans that vegan food can be every bit as delicious as meat or fish dishes.

Above all, and this is something which pretty much every vegan apart from the extremely radical and/or judgemental ones will tell you, don't worry about being perfect and making mistakes. No one's the first and everyone does the second. 'Don't feel that you've failed if you have a slip-up or two – it happens to all of us, and it doesn't mean that you're not a vegan any more. As long as you keep trying, you're still making a difference. Even if you decide to just eat vegan occasionally each week, your choice will lessen the demand for animal produce. Remember also that every time you pick a vegan option when you're out and about, you are influencing the people around you. Depending on your current diet, you could save between 100 and 200 animals every year by going vegan.'[40]

40 Peters, ibid.

'Of all the creatures, man is the most detestable. Of the entire brood, he's the one that possesses malice. He is the only creature that inflicts pain for sport, knowing it to be pain. The fact that man knows right from wrong proves his intellectual superiority to the other creatures; but the fact that he can do wrong proves his moral inferiority to any creature that cannot.'

Mark Twain

KNOW YOUR ONIONS: MYTHS AND OBJECTIONS

This chapter is Bluffer Central: a comprehensive (well, reasonably so, at least that's the hope) guide to 25 common objections to veganism, and how to refute them. As with *Turning over A New Leaf*, forewarned is forearmed. Picture the bluffer as a batsman facing hostile bowling, where the bowlers are those who object to veganism, the stumps are the honour of veganism itself, and the batsman's own skill is all that stands between one and the other. (This may have come to the author in a vegan cheese-prompted dream, perhaps not unconnected to the fact that the Ashes were taking place at the time of writing.) Here, the bat does not say Woodworm, Kookaburra, Gray-Nicolls and so on. Here, the bat only says 'Bluff', and as any aspiring cricketer knows, any good shot always shows the maker's name to the bowler.

A good starting point is the four 'N's of meat-eating: it's natural, necessary, nice and normal.

1. Eating meat is natural

This falls down on three grounds.

First, whether something is natural or not does not in itself render that thing good or bad. Indeed, much of Western civilisation (at this point the bluffer may like to drop in Gandhi's probably apocryphal zinger when asked what he thought of Western civilisation: 'I think it would be a very good idea) is explicitly based on suppressing the individual's natural tendencies, particularly the less palatable ones involving violence, in the interests of social harmony and progress. Most of what we do these days is not natural. It's not natural to drive a car or take a plane or work at a computer, but we do them anyway.

Second, there's not much that's natural about much of the meat we do eat. *Peas of Mind* detailed some of the ways in which chickens, cows and pigs are pumped full of growth-inducing drugs to maximise their capacity to provide meat and minimise their useful lifespan.

Finally, eating meat may be natural to many animals, but a quick look at human anatomy and physiology suggests that the same does not hold true for us. A lion, for example, eats meat because it is a predatory carnivore which will perish if it does not find sufficient prey. To this end, a lion is equipped with the natural tools to hunt that prey: the speed to run it down, the strength to subdue it, the sharpness of teeth and claw to rip it apart into manageable chunks, and a digestive system which can deal with the bacteria in raw meat.

Humans have none of these things. That's why we have supermarkets. Yes, technically we have canine teeth the way carnivores do, but just as critics of Theresa May accused her proposed Brexit withdrawal agreement as being BRINO (Brexit In Name Only), so are our teeth CINO (Canine In Name Only). Or, to take a political example from across the pond, 'fake canines'.

True carnivores have long, sharp, curved canines, as much knife blades as teeth. Our teeth can just about cope with a Big Mac. They are pretty good at breaking apart and chewing vegetables, fruits, nuts, seeds and the like, though. Our teeth are flat and grinding, and our jaws move from side to side. Both of these are very rare among true carnivores, who don't need flat teeth as they don't chew their food and don't need lateral flexibility in their jaws as it increases the possibility of injury.

Nor can we kill any animals other than very small ones (birds and rodents) without using outside implements: a club, gun, knife, rock, trap or similar. We need tools to dismember the carcass, and we have to cook meat thoroughly to minimise the chances of illness and infection. Our intestines are long and folding, forcing food to move slowly through our digestive systems and therefore allowing our bodies to absorb as many nutrients as possible during the process. True carnivores have short intestines to process meat quickly before pathogens in it can be absorbed into their bloodstream through the gut, and they also have very strong stomach acid to help with this (less than 1 on the PH scale, where humans and other plant-eating animals have stomach acid of between 4 and 5).

If all this still doesn't convince the recalcitrant non-bluffer, the bluffer can surely win the point by acidly observing that you don't see lions huddled round a camp fire drinking cheap lager and telling each other ghost stories while they wait for the antelope to be cooked all the way through, do you?

2. Eating meat is necessary
The entire section *Salad Gold* is a direct refutation of this. It could be cut and pasted in here, but that would be a cheap way of padding out the word count and the eagle-eyed editor would (a) notice and (b) be displeased.

3. Eating meat is nice
This is true, for many people, and is one of the main reasons why vegan food companies are investing so much time, effort and money in developing meat-free versions of favourite dishes such as burgers (*see Romaines to be Seen.*)

The sensual allure of meat – taste, smell and texture – plays into one of the complications of veganism: that it is by definition a social choice as well as an individual one. Foer puts it very well when he says that 'our decisions about food are complicated by the fact that we don't eat alone. Table fellowship has forged social bonds as far back as the archaeological record allows us to look. Food, family, and memory are primordially linked. We are not merely animals that eat, but eating animals. Some of my fondest memories are of weekly sushi dinners with my best friend, and eating my dad's turkey burgers with mustard and grilled onions at backyard celebrations, and tasting the salty gefilte fish at my grandmother's house every Passover.

These occasions simply aren't the same without those foods – and that matters. To give up the taste of sushi or roasted chicken is a loss that extends beyond giving up a pleasurable eating experience. Changing what we eat and letting tastes fade from memory create a kind of cultural loss, a forgetting.

'Food is not rational. Food is culture, habit, and identity. For some, that irrationality leads to a kind of resignation. Food choices are likened to fashion choices or lifestyle preferences – they do not respond to judgments about how we should live. And I would agree that the messiness of food, the almost infinite meanings it proliferates, does make the question of eating – and eating animals especially – surprisingly fraught. Activists I spoke with were endlessly puzzled and frustrated by the disconnect between clear thinking and people's food choices. I sympathize, but I also wonder if it is precisely the irrationality of food that holds the most promise.'[41]

Of course, the fact that something is nice does not necessarily make it right. And one of the central tenets of veganism is that the most delicious food in the world will still taste totally unpalatable when you factor in the process by which that food has made its way to your plate.

4. Eating meat is normal
It's only normal because society has, over many decades, made it so. The bluffer can point out that society makes lots of things normal, and if they always stayed that way

41 Foer, ibid.

then nothing would ever change. Societies of yesteryear happily and legally carried out practices which to our modern eyes seem abhorrent (slavery, indigenous genocide, denying women the right to vote, outlawing homosexuality, and so on).

The 'normality' argument works along the same lines as 'If eating meat was wrong, the government would ban it.' There's a big difference between legality and morality, and there's an equally big difference between state proscription and individual responsibility. Governments are not, and most people would argue should not be, the ultimate arbiters of morality; morality is a personal issue, and everyone's moral framework is slightly different.

There are certain things which every civilised society believes are beyond the pale – murder and rape being two of the most obvious examples – and they are both outlawed and subject to the severest sanctions available under the relevant legal code. Eating meat is not seen by most of society as even in the same ballpark as those crimes, though of course in decades and centuries to come this may change (*see Romaines to be Seen*). In addition, government legislation is heavily influenced by the lobbying efforts of powerful commercial interests who are more concerned with money than morality (the bluffer can point out that the only two absolute imperatives incumbent on any commercial enterprise are to maximise shareholder revenue and remain within the bounds of the law).

Now let's throw the conversation open to the floor. You, sir. No, not you. You. Yes, in the blue shirt. Speak right into the microphone, please.

s would survive the way they have done
sands of years.

vent vegan, farmers and slaughter-
would lose their jobs

's not going to go vegan overnight, so
his area will be gradual. But the more
egan, the more job opportunities there
egan food sector, so these farmers and
ill almost certainly be able to find work
arket never remains static: new sectors
even as old ones are made obsolete. Just
ing (in this case, meat) is available for
n that consumers are obliged to buy it.
eryone would smoke and drink in order
in those industries gainfully employed.

feel pain, too

tional understanding available to us
ientific knowledge they can't, as plants
tral nervous system. The bluffer's vast
nowledge of literature will include the
ld Dahl did write a short story called
e about a man who invents a machine
lants screaming, but then again he also
iant flying peach and a glass elevator
through space without even a vaguely
on system, so it isn't really necessary
lves too much with his commitment to
cy. Even if we could prove that plants
hat would still reinforce rather than

5. My grandmother ate a full English breakfast every day and lived to be 114

Good for her. This does not in and of itself prove that veganism is unnecessary for good health, and it certainly doesn't prove that eating full Englishes day in day out is good for you. The only thing it proves is that your grandmother had the constitution of an ox. Individual anecdotes, as the bluffer well knows, are not in and of themselves acceptable scientific evidence. Not all smokers develop lung cancer, and not everyone who does develop lung cancer is a smoker, but the causal link between cigarettes and lung cancer has now been established beyond any shred of doubt. Any decent scientific study must be run within strictly controlled parameters, across a population sample wide enough to account for individual variation, and with rigorous attention to statistical analysis.

6. If you were on a desert island and you had to eat meat to survive, you'd do it

Well, not only is this is a strictly hypothetical and vanishingly unlikely scenario, but even if it happened – and actually plenty of vegans would literally prefer to die than take another animal's life – it would not invalidate the central tenets of veganism. There's a huge difference between killing out of necessity (as some subsistence hunters do to this day) and out of choice, and this is before factoring in the life conditions of the animal in question rather than just the manner of its death.

People do extreme things when they're faced with pure questions of survival, but they don't take that kind of behaviour back into normal life with them. The Uruguayan survivors of the 1972 Andes plane crash ate flesh from the dead bodies of their fellow passengers, but they didn't subsequently ask to see the cannibal options on the menu of their favourite Montevideo restaurants.

The desert island question also falls down on moral and practical grounds. If we're going to judge the worth of any given ideology purely on whether or not one would give one's life for it, we're not going to find much left to believe in (and of course the converse is true: that suicide bombers give their lives for a cause doesn't in and of itself make that cause worthy, at least not to the vast majority of society). And in practical terms, if there are animals on this desert island then there are almost certainly plants for them to eat, so you could just eat those instead.

(If the desert island in question is the Radio 4 one with discs attached, however, you'll be in Broadcasting House just north of Oxford Street where there are plenty of vegan-friendly establishments within walking distance, unless it has recently turned into a wild and lawless place full of nature red in tooth and claw. Rather like Oxford Circus tube station at rush hour, come to think of it.)

7. A friend turned vegan and had health problems as a result

A slam dunk for the bluffer here, who can point out that your friend didn't have health problems as a result of turning vegan: they had problems either because they

failed to eat a bala
because they had
to their lifestyle
properly planned
anyone needs, wit
which can easily

8. If everyone tu
take over the w
The author has in
Apocalypse Cow (o
decided yet) in wl
grids, and from th
bowing low befor
unsurprisingly, He
this one. You can

Farm animals
everyone turns v
exist in such hug
overbred for food
animals would set
lower quantities
going to go vegan
would be gradual

An equal and
turned vegan, fa
Some farm anim
But they would
full of predators
as nature inten
conditions of fac

that each specie
for tens of thou

9. If everyone
house workers
Again, everyone
any change in t
people who go
will be in the v
other workers w
there. The job m
come to the fore
because someth
sale doesn't mea
By that logic, ev
to keep workers

10. Plants can
Not by any ra
under current so
don't have a cer
and extensive k
nugget that Ro
The Sound Machi
which can hear
wrote about a
which travelled
feasible propuls
to concern ours
scientific accura
did feel pain,

undermine the cause of veganism, as animals raised for food eat far more plants than we do.

11. If we didn't milk cows, their udders would explode

Leaving aside the image of various cattle ending up like Monty Python's Mr Creosote – no, they wouldn't explode, but they would become very distended and painful – this demonstrates not just a misunderstanding of bovine physiology but also a very human-centric way of looking at things. Cows don't produce milk for humans. They produce milk for their calves, who are forcibly separated from their mothers immediately after birth. If the calves were allowed to stay with the mothers and drink the milk (they suckle naturally every 20 minutes or so) there would be no problem. And cows, like most mammals, only lactate after giving birth and/ or when nursing their young.

12. The farm animals are going to be killed anyway

In narrow technical terms, this is true. But they're only going to be killed anyway for the same specific reason they were born and raised in the first place – that there's consumer demand for them. Remove that demand and the killing will stop.

13. Most farms are not factory farms

The actual numbers of farms are less important than the fact that the vast majority of animals are born, live and die on factory farms. If you have ten farms, one of which is a factory farm holding 5,000 cows and the other nine are smallholdings with 50 cows each, only 10% of the farms will be factory, but more than 90% of the cows will be kept in factory conditions. (GCSE maths questions have changed a bit since the 1970s, that's for sure.)

See also 'I only buy free-range', and *see Peas of Mind* for what 'free-range' actually means.

14. What about pets? You feed your pets meat, don't you? And you have your pets put down. What's the difference?

Two questions in one there, but that's what happens when you need to keep these points down to a round 25.

First things first. Yes, vegans do feed their pets meat, because most pets, particularly dogs and cats, need meat in a way that humans don't. There are meat-free pet food companies out there to help reduce pets' carbon pawprints, and these companies' products do contain protein, but they also need to contain the correct amino acids within that protein, and that can be hard on a non-meat diet. As things stand, it's very difficult – read: in practical terms, all but impossible – to give your pets no meat whatsoever and still stay within official nutritional guidelines (and failing to do the latter can potentially lead to owners being charged under the Animal Welfare Act). Veganism is about the best interests of the animal in question rather than merely the moral viewpoint of the owner, and therefore feeding your pet non-vegan food is logically consistent.

As for putting pets down: you put a pet down when

it's suffering, when it has little or no quality of life, and when the vet tells you there's no hope of recovery. When you do decide to go down this route, you almost always stay with your pet while the anaesthetic takes effect, and only when the animal is unconscious does the vet administer a lethal injection. There's literally no comparison between that and an animal which is force-fed, kept in cramped conditions, can expect to survive only a fraction of its natural lifespan, and stands a good chance of being conscious or semi-conscious when its throat is cut in a loud, terrifying slaughterhouse.

15. We are more intelligent than animals and therefore have the right to use them how we see fit

Intelligence is no measure of the worth of any life (a hard one for the bluffer to swallow, granted, but bear with us). By that logic, people with higher IQs would arrogate themselves the right to choose how to treat those with lower IQs. Man's intellectual capacity to do things has always run some way behind his moral capacity to decide whether or not to do those things.

16. Veganism is a personal choice. You have no right to tell others what to do

It is a personal choice, yes: a choice which was denied to the animals killed for their meat. As for telling others what to do – well, this is a free country, and everyone's entitled not just to hold an opinion but also to express it (other than the obvious ones which break the law, such as incitement to racial hatred or daring to suggest that *Fleabag* is anything other than a work of staggering genius). By the same token, everyone's entitled to heed or ignore those opinions. (On a tactical level, as discussed in *Cool Beans*, most vegans have realised that persuasion so gentle as to be almost unnoticeable is preferable to hectoring in the loudest and most strident voice since the original hectoring – viz., Achilles, aka Brad Pitt standing by the walls of Troy and shouting 'Hector! Hectooooooor!')

'How do you know if someone's vegan? Don't worry. They'll tell you.'

---

17. Vegans are self-righteous

Hence the oldest joke in the vegan book: 'How do you know if someone's vegan? Don't worry. They'll tell you.' Yes, some vegans are self-righteous. So are some non-vegans. And though that may (understandably) make them irritating, it doesn't by extension make them wrong.

Bluffers, whether vegan or non-vegan, are never self-righteous, of course, and how very dare anyone who suggests otherwise.

18. If you think eating meat is immoral, you must think that all meat-eaters are immoral too

Not at all. Meat-eating is an immoral cultural practice, but it's so entrenched and ingrained in our culture that many millions of good people do it without thinking too much about the issue.

19. Vegans damage the planet in other ways

We all damage the planet in some way; it's an inevitable by-product of existing. And yes, plenty of vegans could take shorter showers, fewer car journeys and so on (though vegans are in general and for obvious reasons fairly well attuned to environmental issues). But pointing out someone's flaws in other areas to distract from their primary message is classic 'whataboutery'.

20. I'm too busy and don't have time to learn a whole new way of eating

The initial learning-curve can be steep and time-consuming, true, but it soon becomes second nature. And – this is not confined to veganism, by any means – 'I don't have time' more often than not means 'I don't regard it as a priority'/'I can't be arsed.' People make time for what's important to them.

21. Veganism is a first world luxury

It's true that first world diets have range and balance denied to many people in developing countries. But global animal agriculture affects developing countries quite as much as it does developed ones: deforestation for soya production, for instance (more than 90% of soya goes to feed animals rather than humans), and the widespread use of immigrants to work in slaughterhouses.

22. Veganism is a white middle-class thing

It's true that the majority of vegan influencers and authors are white and middle class, but the same is true across pretty much every media sector. (BAME under-representation is a real problem, but also one way outside the scope of this book.) There is no reason why veganism should be confined to any one race, colour or class. A vegan diet doesn't have to be any more expensive than a non-vegan one; in fact, given the cost of meat, it may well end up being cheaper.

23. The whole world will never be vegan

The bluffer can do a classic bait-and-switch here by admitting that this is almost certainly true – and then, when the non-bluffer is preening themself at having finally got one over the bluffer, the bluffer can calmly point out that the world will also almost certainly never be free of racism, sexism, homophobia and other prejudices, let alone violence and inequality. That's no reason either to stop fighting against those things or indeed to actively practise them.

The bluffer may or may not want to sign off this argument with a 'chef's kiss' (kissing the fingertips before opening them and withdrawing the hand in a way that indicates sublime deliciousness). A vegan chef's kiss, of course.

24. You can't be 100% vegan in modern society, so why bother?

Yes, animal products are used in so many different places and ways that it's almost impossible to live totally free from them. That's why the Vegan Society includes the phrase 'as far as is possible and practicable' in its mission to exclude 'all forms of exploitation of, and cruelty to, animals for food, clothing or any other purpose'.

Veganism isn't about trying to be perfect, but living in a way which does the least possible harm – and, as more and more people become vegan, their critical consumerist mass will prompt companies and innovators to develop increasingly animal-free alternatives to current methods of production. Companies operate on what might be termed 'enlightened self-interest'; that is, they are most minded to do moral good when there's a commercial upside to it too.

Turning vegan won't save the animals currently in the slaughterhouses, but a lifetime of veganism equates to a possible 10,000 uneaten animals, and when demand decreases so does supply.

---

25. One person can't make a difference

This is a self-fulfilling prophecy. If everyone accepted the status quo as it is, then of course things will never change. The only way to make a difference is to change the one thing over which you have responsibility – yourself. Turning vegan won't save the animals currently in the slaughterhouses, but a lifetime of veganism equates to a possible 10,000 uneaten animals, and when demand decreases so does supply.

Then there's the domino effect of inspiring others to

make the change. There are plenty of vegan communities, and with every new member they gain a tiny bit more traction and influence. As the cultural anthropologist Margaret Mead said: 'Never doubt that a small group of thoughtful, committed citizens can change the world; indeed, it's the only thing that ever has.'

I HERB IT THROUGH THE GRAPEVINE

It's not just in the UK that veganism is on the rise. Similar trends can be seen across much of the developed world, and plenty of cities which the vegan traveller might find themselves visiting boast widespread vegan restaurants, supermarkets and other resources. (Cities are, as noted in *Kale of Duty*, in general more vegan-friendly than rural areas.)

The bluffer, of course, need not even have visited these cities, let alone tried out anything remotely vegan there. The crucial thing is that he can loftily claim to have done so, and inform his interlocutors that they 'simply must visit this darling little place in New York/Paris/Tel Aviv, the vegan food is *divine*. It's a little off the beaten track, of course, but all the better for that. Always eat where the locals do, eh?'

So without further ado, let's go round the world in quite a lot less than 80 vegan days (that is, in 10 vegan cities, organised strictly alphabetically), and give you a few names to memorise and drop into the conversation at opportune moments.

AMSTERDAM

Amsterdam is no stranger to the herb, so veganism is a fairly logical extension of that, no? Hummus House is the latest in the series of 'does what it says on the tin', *TerraZen Central* fuses Caribbean and Japanese cuisine (fried tempeh and avocado sushi, anyone?), and *Men Impossible* does all-vegan ramen.

BERLIN

Given its history as a counterculture hub during the Cold War and current hipness, it's no surprise that Berlin has a thriving and growing vegan scene. (Germany accounted for 15% of global vegan product launches between July 2017 and June 2018, more than any other country.)[42] Perhaps the heart of vegan Berlin is *Schivelbeiner Straße*, also known as 'Vegan Avenue', which boasts the vegan shoe store *Avesu*, the vegan clothing store *Deargoods*, and the *Veganz* vegan grocery store (plus café, naturally). But vegan outlets can be found across the city and cater for a wide variety of tastes: vegan pizzas at *La Stella Nera*, vegan doner kebab at *Vöner der Vegetarische Döner*, gourmet cuisine at *Lucky Leek*, raw food at, er, *Rawtastic*, and a plethora of Asian

42 Mintel report, 2018.

vegan restaurants. You can even get a vegan tattoo at *Lightworkers.*

LOS ANGELES

Well, of *course* LA's going to be a vegan-friendly city. Hollywood, baby! There are plenty of ethnic vegan options: Thai restaurants such as *Arraya's Place* and *Satdha*, Ethiopian (*Rahel, Azla*), upscale Japanese (*Shojin*), Vietnamese (*Au Lac*), and Cuban (*Equelecua*). *Vromage* does vegan cheese and *Cruzer* vegan pizza. Vegan musician Moby owns the *Little Pine* bistro (Italian/Mediterranean fusion). *Donut Farm, Bakery LA* and *Pomegranate* are all good vegan bakeries, and *Moo Shoes* sells vegan shoes and accessories.

NEW YORK CITY

New York was once and is still arguably the food capital of the world – it's certainly up there in contention for that accolade – and this applies every bit as much to vegan cuisine as non-vegan. *Terri's* is a good chain with outlets across the city, either under its own name or that of *P.S. Kitchen. Marty's V Burger* has vegan burgers and buffalo wings – hey! It's New York. What do you expect? – and further up the gourmet (and price) spectrum are *Blossom* and *Candle 79*. Ethnic vegan outlets include *Hangawi* (Korean/Asian fusion) and *Delice & Sarrasin* (French crepes). Also in the category of HINY (Hey! It's New York) are vegan confectionery store *Confectionery!* (seriously, guys? All that brand consulting and marketing spend and you just shove an exclamation mark on the end of what you sell?) and vegan doughnut bakery *Dun-Well Doughnuts* (for the clean-eating cop on a stakeout, as seen in roughly 19,834 films set in New York since the dawn of cinema).

PARIS

You may not instantly associate veganism with French cuisine – this is, after all, the nation which brings you both escargots and foie gras – but perhaps it's inevitable that in a city of Paris's size and culinary history there'll be plenty of vegan options. *Gentle Gourmet* does classical and contemporary refined cuisine, *Hank Vegan Burger* serves what many consider the best vegan burger in the city, and its sister restaurant *Hank Vegan Pizza* is well regarded too. *Le Potager Du Marais* serves vegan twists on traditional French foods such as bourguinon, and *My Kitch'n* serves a vegan version of foie gras called faux gras (punning worthy of the *Bluffer's Guide* itself there). For vegan Vietnamese food, check out *La Palanche d'Aulac*. *Super Vegan's* kebab with garlic sauce is justifiably famous among aficionados, and both *Hot Vog* and *Le Tricycle* offer vegan hot dogs. *Cloud Cakes*, *Jo & Nana Cakes*, *Laélo* and *VG Pâtisserie* all sell vegan desserts, cakes and ice cream. *Un Monde Vegan* and *Mon Epicerie Paris* are both good vegan groceries, *Jay & Joy* specialises in vegan cheese, and *Veganie* sells several brands of vegan cosmetics.

PORTLAND

Portland, Oregon, that is, not Portland, Maine, and certainly not Portland across the causeway from Weymouth on Dorset's Jurassic Coast. Portland has long been exactly the kind of trendy progressive north-western city (hipsters, cyclists, craft beers) where you'd expect to find a wide array of vegan resources, and it doesn't disappoint – there's even a totally vegan shopping mall. Almost every restaurant offers some kind of plant-based option, and there are plenty of dedicated vegan places too. *Vtopia Cheese Shop & Deli* sells 20 types of vegan artisanal cheese, which is roughly 19 more types than most people knew existed. In the same building is the *Ichiza Kitchen and Teahouse*, which offers Buddhist cuisine. Fans of vegan Israeli food can go to *Aviv*; *Homegrown Smoker* caters for vegan barbecuers (and now that cannabis is legal in Oregon they could branch out into that market too without needing to bother with a name change); *Virtuous Pie* has good pizzas if the slight smuggery of the name doesn't put you off; vegan Peruvian food is all yours at *Paiche*; *Back to Eden*, which is exclusively vegan and gluten-free, is widely held up as the best bakery/sweet shop in the city; and *Blossoming Lotus* offers fine vegan dining (the bluffer can go all misty-eyed when 'remembering' the almond ricotta bruschetta and roasted delicate squash tacos). Portland even has several adult entertainment clubs serving only vegan food, so you can help save the planet even while reneging on your marriage vows (there must be some form of cosmic balancing equation there, but we don't have the time or frankly the maths skills to work it out). Non-food vegan outlets include *Ether Shoes Warehouse* (which sells clothing and accessories too), *Herbivore Clothing* and the *New Moon Massage* vegan massage therapy studio.

PRAGUE

If eastern European cuisine conjures up visions of heavy meat and dairy stodge, nothing could be further from the truth, at least in Prague. It has among the highest number of vegan restaurants per capita of any city in the world. A few years ago, the city's vegan scene more or less began and ended with the *Loving Hut* chain, but now the discerning vegan can find local cuisine at *Bistro Střecha* (which is owned by a worker's co-operative and offers jobs to former prisoners and the homeless among others). *Chlebíček* sells typical Czech open sandwiches, *Forrest Bistro* mixes and matches several different national cuisines, and both *Waipawa Letná* and *Pastva* offer vegan burgers. *Amitabha* does vegan Thai food, *bistRAWveg* caters for raw food, and the *Blue Vegan Pig Shop* sells doughnuts.

TEL AVIV

Israel has the highest number of vegans per capita in the world: one in every 20 Israelis is vegan,[43] and the lifestyle is both widely accepted and deeply entrenched

---

43 *The Culture Trip*, January 2019.

in the culture (the Israeli Defence Force provides vegan soldiers not just with vegan meals but also leather-free boots and helmets).

The usual reasons aside, there are several factors behind veganism's popularity in Israel. (This is prime bluffer's territory, right at the intersection of politics, religion and cultural anthropology: a mini-dissertation entitled *Popular Attitudes towards Plant-based Dietary Frameworks in the Levant*.)

Vegan promoter Ori Shavit says that 'Israel is a nation of immigrants that came from all over the world with their own cultures and cuisines. The country is very young and still evolving so people here are less attached to traditional eating, they are used to trying new things and love innovations – therefore they are less scared to make a change in their diet.' Since many Jewish Israelis are used to keeping kosher, they 'are familiar with the idea of thinking before they eat, checking the ingredients, looking at the label, avoiding certain foods and separating others'.

Animal protection activist Ondine Sherman also credits politics with promoting veganism, albeit inadvertently. 'Many young Israelis feel disempowered and despondent by years of stagnation and lack of progress towards peace [with Palestine]. Animal rights and vegan activism are social justice movements where each individual can make a direct positive impact on the lives of animals. Making a difference, being a force for change, is empowering and invigorating.'

The national cuisine is to a large extent plant-based

anyway, and so it stands to reason that Tel Aviv boasts a cornucopia of vegan restaurants. *Tenat* is a well-regarded all-vegan Ethiopian restaurant, *Zakaim* is a farm-to-table outlet which grows all its own food (bluffer tip: burnt aubergine with tahini and homemade challah bread), and *Four One Six* is a modern New York-style bar and restaurant. *The Green Roll* does vegan sushi, *Rawfood* does what it says on the tin, *Falafel Mevorach* serves vegan kebabs, shawarma, schnitzel and burgers, and *Hatool HaYarok* does vegan pizza with cashew cheese. *Taam L'Chaim* – Taste for Life – is a vegan grocery store.

TORONTO

The Toronto Veg Food Fest has long been one of North America's largest vegetarian events, so it's not surprising that plenty of establishments have gone one step further and become vegan. *Apiecalypse Now* is a vegan pizzeria, *Mythology Diner* features vegan versions of classic diner foods, and both *Urban Herbivore* and *Kupfert & Kim* offer create-it-yourself vegan protein bowl restaurants. *Planta* has upscale vegan dining covered, *Vegetarian Haven* features Asian fusion cuisine, and Jamaican vegan food can be found at *One Love Vegetarian* and *Ital Vital*. *Rawlicious* is – well, you're getting the hang of this by now, aren't you? – and *Sweet Hart Kitchen* caters for vegan desserts. *The Good Rebel* is a vegan grocery store, and *Imperative* sells vegan shirts, shoes, purses, wallets, and accessories.

WARSAW

The city is sprouting vegan restaurants at an almost exponential rate, and since most of them are in or near the city centre they're mainly within walking distance of each other. *Vege Miasto*, *Lokal Vegan Bistro* and *Vege Bistro* all serve vegan versions of traditional Polish dishes such as *pierogi* (dumplings), *golabki* (cabbage rolls) and *schabowy* (meat cutlets). *Krowarzywa*, which has four outlets, has twice been voted as having the 'Best Burger in Warsaw' – not just the best vegan burger, you understand, but the best burger full stop, beating out the entire meat-based competition. *Edamame* and *Youmiko* offer vegan sushi; *Leonardo Verde* is Italian; *Keboom* offers vegan kebabs; and the *Vegan Ramen Shop* is fairly self-explanatory, as are *FalafeLove* and *Falafel Beirut*. *Akwarium* and *Vegestacja* offer vegan ice cream, and *Lokal Dela Krem* serves cakes and other baked goods. Warsaw also has two vegan grocery stores, *Evergreen* and *TerraVege*; a vegan wine shop, *Solvino Bio*; a vegan shoe store, *Amanas*; and two vegan nail salons, *Salon Wisla* and *Nailed It*.

'One of the amazing effects that going vegan has on our bodies is changing the way we smell and taste – and all for the better.'

PETA

SOWING OATS: VEGANISM AND SEX

Few areas of life are immune from the effects of sex, and the bluffer will know that veganism is no different.

For a start, it's widely claimed (mainly by vegans, naturally) that vegans make better lovers. A pre-Valentine's Day article on the PETA website says that 'many vegan foods boost blood circulation – including to the brain, which has a positive effect on the libido. Eating these foods actually improves circulation to all parts of the body, so we have a much higher chance of getting the results we're looking for in the bedroom. It's simple: increased blood circulation = better physical response = better sex. Stock up on cayenne pepper, leafy greens, figs, pumpkin seeds, dark chocolate, and almonds – great sources of vitamin B and zinc, which elevate testosterone levels and sexual desire.

'One of the amazing effects that going vegan has on our bodies is changing the way we smell and taste – and all for the better. A 2006 study on body odour found that people eating plant-based food smelled significantly better than those eating meat, while some people say that when men eat vegan meals packed with fruits and veggies, [*warning! adult content ahead*] their semen tastes sweeter.'[44]

This is genius-level marketing, of course: take the demographic traditionally most resistant to veganism (men), home in on the main reason for their resistance (the equation between meat and virility), and flip that on its head by telling them that going vegan will actually improve their sex life; that vegans are virile and carnivores castrated. 'Consuming low-fat vegan meals can help combat the most common causes of impotence: high cholesterol, obesity, diabetes, prostate cancer or inflammation, and hormonal imbalances. A study published in *The American Journal of Clinical Nutrition* suggests that men who couple regular exercise with a diet rich in flavonoids, found in fruits like strawberries, blueberries, and apples, may reduce their risk of developing erectile dysfunction by over 20 per cent.'[45]

The Oscar-winning director James Cameron agrees (the bluffer should of course frame this as an airy 'Cameron agrees', thus implying that one is on intimate terms with one of the premier film-makers of the age (and indeed leaving open the tantalising possibility that one might also be referring to the erstwhile Prime Minister and architect of a referendum which has in no way had political repercussions). In the 2018 documentary *The*

44 www.peta.org.uk, February 2019.
45 www.peta.org.uk, ibid.

Game Changers, which Cameron executive produced, one scene (which Cameron calls the 'peter meter' scene) shows three men having the length and girth of their erections measured after eating plant-based meals – and all three experienced better erections. 'I'd love to put Viagra out of business, just by spreading the word on plant-based eating,' Cameron said in a newspaper interview to promote his production.[46]

However, many scientists say that insufficient studies on a causal link between a vegan diet and increased sexual stamina have been carried out, and point out that plenty of non-vegan foods aid a good sex life, including salmon (the omega-3 fatty acids trigger arousal) and chicken breast (Vitamin B aids erectile tissue).

More generally, a vegan lifestyle plays out in various ways when it comes to sex. There are now increasing numbers of vegan sex aids such as condoms (including those made by the German company Einhorn; who says the Germans have no sense of humour?), lubricants and sex toys.

Whether or not vegans get to use these with non-vegans is a different matter. PETA's founder and president Ingrid Newkirk thinks sex is the best way of converting non-vegans to the cause. 'When my staff members come to me and say: 'Guess what? My boyfriend, now he's a vegan,' I say, half-jokingly: "Well, it is time to ditch him and get another. You've done your work; move on."'[47] But research on online dating sites

46 *Toronto Star*, April 2018.
47 *New York Times*, December 2007.

has found that the more someone enjoys eating meat, the less likely they are to swipe right on a vegan.[48] Also, the connection between meat-eating and masculinity mentioned above means that some women find vegan men less attractive than those who eat meat.[49]

Of course, it works the other way too. In what can sometimes seem, particularly to the older and more traditional bluffer, a world of increasing sexual fluidity, it should come as no surprise that some vegans identify as 'vegansexual'; that is, they are either more attracted to other vegans than to non-vegans, or they will refuse to sleep with anybody other than their fellow vegans.

In her unimprovably titled study *Vegan Sexuality: Challenging Heteronormative Masculinity through Meat-free Sex*,[50] New Zealand researcher Annie Potts recorded vegan survey respondents as reluctant to become romantically involved with non-vegans for several reasons: 'I couldn't think of kissing lips that allow dead animal pieces to pass between them'; 'Non-vegetarian bodies smell different to me. They are, after all, literally sustained through carcasses – the murdered flesh of others'; and an unbridgeably wide gulf in 'shared values and moral codes'.

48 'What's your beef with vegetarians? Predicting anti-vegetarian prejudice from pro-beef attitudes across cultures.' Earle and Hodson, *Personality and Individual Differences*, 2016.
49 'Eating meat makes you sexy: conformity to dietary gender norms and attractiveness.' Timeo and Suitner, *Psychology of Men & Masculinity*, 2018.
50 Annie Potts and Jovian Parry, *Feminism & Psychology*, 2010.

ROMAINES TO BE SEEN: THE FUTURE OF VEGANISM

The bluffer can hint at many hours spent in top-level investment meetings by opining that the vegan industry is undergoing substantial and seismic change, and will continue to do so; not just in terms of the numbers as an increasing amount of people become vegan, but also in terms of innovation, research and development.

In September 2019, the first vegan exchange-traded fund (ETF) was launched on the New York Stock Exchange. The US Vegan Climate ETF has pledged 'not to invest in companies that harm animals, and screens out firms that farm animals, make food from them or use them for entertainment'. While the fund is not the first to pick stocks according to a strict environmental or ethical rulebook, it is the first ETF to be marketed as being completely vegan. It does this by tracking a vetted index made by Beyond Investing – the same vegan and cruelty-free investment platform that runs the new fund.[51]

HALO EFFECT

Giant food companies are already moving in on the vegan sector, either by creating vegan lines of their own (often as 'halo' products for the rest of their range), investing in (or buying outright) smaller vegan firms, or both. Greggs' vegan sausage roll is among the chain's top five bestselling items, and was launched amid a blaze of social media publicity (no doubt helped by the fact that the TV presenter Piers Morgan hated it: 'Nobody was waiting for a vegan sausage, you PC-ravaged clowns,' he tweeted).[52] The success prompted Greggs' CEO Roger Whiteside to tell LBC radio in August 2019 that 'we are working away to see if we can come up with a [vegan] version of all our bestselling lines because people want vegan options. If we can produce something that tastes just as good as the meat version, then that will sell very successfully. That's what's been shown with the vegan sausage roll.'

At the beginning of 2018 McDonald's launched the McVegan burger in a limited number of outlets in Sweden and Finland. In December 2018 Unilever bought The Vegetarian Butcher, a Dutch meat-substitute company. Tyson Foods, one of the largest meat companies in the US, has a 5% stake in Beyond Meat, an alternative meat

51 *Daily Telegraph*, September 2019.
52 *The Guardian*, September 2019.

company which in May 2019 floated on the NASDAQ exchange valued at $3.8bn (and which was valued at $11.7bn two months later).

ALTERNATIVE MEAT

Beyond Meat makes and sells vegan meat substitutes – Beyond Chicken, Beyond Beef, Beyond Sausage, the Beast Burger – made from mixtures of pea protein isolates, rice protein, mung bean protein, canola oil, coconut oil, and other ingredients like potato starch, apple extract, sunflower lecithin, and pomegranate powder with a range of vitamins and minerals. Beet juice is used to mimic the 'bleeding' of real meat.

Beyond Meat and rival companies are in the vanguard of the alternative meat market; that is, vegan products designed to mimic the look, feel and taste of meat without, of course, containing any actual meat. But this is only one-half of the potential market.

CLEAN MEAT

The other is 'clean meat'; that is, actual meat which is grown in a laboratory from animal cells, and therefore does not involve the slaughter (and, by extension, the mistreatment) of any animals. (Knowing and expounding on the difference between 'clean' and 'alternative' meat is an excellent way for the bluffer to hint at serious knowledge in an obscure field, which is after all why we're here.)

'We start with high-quality animal cells,' said

David Kay, head of mission and business analyst for Memphis Meats. 'We feed those cells nutrients (water, sugars, proteins, fats, vitamins and nutrients): the same macronutrients that cows obtain when they eat grass. Once the cells grow sufficiently, we harvest them and they are ready to be cooked and prepared just like conventionally produced meat. Essentially, we are recreating a process that naturally occurs inside an animal's body, but doing it outside that animal's body.'[53]

'The two big questions an awful lot of the companies are focused on: how do we feed 9bn people by 2050, and how do we address climate change?' said Bruce Friedrich, head of the Good Food Institute (GFI) which supports and lobbies on behalf of meat alternative interests. 'Food tech and clean meat are the answer to both questions. All of the positive nutritional aspects of meat, those will be replicated.'[54] One survey has only 40% of the global population consuming animal meat by 2040, with 35% choosing clean laboratory meat and 25% vegan meat replacements.[55]

The question of animal cruelty apart, clean meat has several other advantages over conventional meat. It could be produced with up to 96% less greenhouse gas emissions, 45% less energy, 99% less land use and 96% less water use.[56] It will make it easier for food scientists to refine and maximise calorific and nutritional yields. And it would eliminate the need for antibiotics in the source

53 www.medium.com, July 2018.
54 www.qz.com, November 2017.
55 A.T. Kearney, 2019.
56 Oxford University Wildlife Conservation Research Unit, 2011.

material, as it will not use any live animals and therefore not have to deal with animal disease and infection.

LAB CULTURE

There are, of course, several drawbacks too. Candace Croney, Professor in the departments of Comparative Pathobiology and Animal Sciences and Director of the Center for Animal Welfare Science at Purdue University, Indiana, USA, says: 'Is growing meat in a laboratory socially acceptable to people? We don't know that yet. People who lean toward "natural" products might have questions about growing meat in a laboratory instead of using more traditional practices. We know many people today are very sensitive about the technologies associated with food production – particularly anything that looks like genetic modification as people tend to be very risk averse. Will this technology be similarly worrisome to people? What information will be provided to the general public here and elsewhere in the world? When and by whom will that be offered so that people can make informed choices that align with their values and beliefs rather than feeling that technology is being foisted on them?

'To the extent that technology advances might make it difficult to economically and visually distinguish cultured meat from traditionally produced meat, will cultured meat products be labelled in such a manner as to facilitate consumer choice? If the products are nutritionally different or vary significantly in price, who will have access to them and how does this mitigate or worsen societal inequities? What happens to rural communities and all the people who are directly or indirectly involved in animal agriculture? It's a way of life that's important to many people. Is it socially acceptable to do something that could disrupt or displace that way of life? As consumers have increasingly expressed a desire to know more about how food is produced and to feel connected to farming, will this type of meat production exacerbate existing tensions and areas of disconnect between those who produce food and those dependent on them as consumers?'[57]

As far as vegans are concerned, would 'clean meat' be acceptable? If it involved no cruelty to animals, had minimal environmental impact and was not detrimental to personal or global health – the three main reasons people give for going vegan – how many vegans would think it acceptable to eat clean meat? It would, after all, still be meat. The answer is, of course, that at this stage we can't possibly tell. (Yes, sometimes the bluffer has to accept limitations to their apparent knowledge.)

There are too many variables; not just the ones we know that we don't yet know, but also the ones we don't know that we don't yet know. (Any resemblance to former US Defence Secretary Donald Rumsfeld's 'known unknowns' is entirely deliberate.) Perhaps the vegan movement would split just as the vegetarian movement did, between those prepared to eat clean meat and those who refuse to.

---

57 www.bestfoodfacts.org, July 2018.

VEGAN WORLD

What would a world look like where that was a realistic choice? What would, in fact, an all-vegan world be

---

As far as vegans are concerned, would 'clean meat' be acceptable? If it involved no cruelty to animals, had minimal environmental impact and was not detrimental to personal or global health – the three main reasons people give for going vegan – how many vegans would think it acceptable to eat clean meat?

---

like: a world where no one ate animal meat (and/or where it was a strictly contraband substance whose consumers – carnists – faced not just long jail sentences but social opprobrium), where no animals were raised to be slaughtered for food, where factory farms were looked upon with the same horror that we view Nazi-era concentration camps, where the word 'veganism' no longer existed as it was simply accepted as the universal norm? Would we all be long, thin, green-tinged and etiolated? (No, sorry: that's Area 51.)

For a start, the environmental impact of an all-vegan

and loss of productivity (though we may of course have the technology to overcome this in the future). Either way, land unsuitability would be offset by a reduction in the amount of farmland needed; scientist Joseph Poore has put the figure at 3.1 billion hectares, more or less the size of Africa,[60] and much of that land could be replanted with trees to help store carbon.

Rural communities in both the developed and developing worlds could find themselves undergoing serious upheaval, since so much of their livelihoods revolve around livestock. This would by no means be insuperable – there would be job opportunities in, for example, reforestation and crop-based bioenergy – but it would need attention to prevent widespread unemployment and even social unrest. The problem would be greatest for nomadic communities who rely on livestock, such as the Mongols of central Asia, the Berbers of North Africa and the Maasai in east Africa. In an all-vegan world they would be forced to relocate to cities to find work, and would lose much if not all of their cultural identity in the process.

60 Oxford University study, 2018.

AMAIZING GRACE: A POSTSCRIPT

There's no point in pretending that you know everything about veganism – nobody does (including the author). But if you've got this far and absorbed at least a modicum of the information and advice contained within these pages, then you will almost certainly know more than 99% of the rest of the human race about the hottest topic in the food world right now. Most importantly, you will know how to pretend to know more about it than you do. What you now do with this information is up to you, but here's a suggestion: be confident about your new-found knowledge, see how far it takes you, but above all, have fun using it. You are now a fully-fledged expert in one of humankind's most valued and unique traditions – the suggestion, artfully disguised and always falling the right side of an outright lie, that you are a world authority on the matter at hand.

Sometimes, however, the bluffer finds that they are

doing things for real. I discovered this myself while writing this book. I wasn't a vegan when I started, but I was by the time I'd finished. It wasn't any one thing which made me change, but a combination – of the three main reasons most people cite, of the mountains of research which I've tried to distil into a relatively small amount of words, of watching undercover videos from factory farms and slaughterhouses, of reading the autobiographies of Scott Jurek and Rich Roll, of talking to friends who are vegan, and so on.

A few days after making the decision, I was at a barbecue. Someone put a chicken on the grill – a dead, washed and prepared chicken, of course, ready to be cooked. I looked at it, and it was like seeing something very familiar with fresh eyes. It looked hideous. I couldn't have brought myself to eat it even if I'd tried. It wasn't a reaction I'd expected to have, and the strength of it rather shook me.

Not long afterwards, I was asked if I had any special dietary requirements for an upcoming function I was due to attend. I was about to reply the same way I'd always replied to such questions – a breezy 'I eat anything' – before realising that actually I don't anymore. Writing 'I'm vegan' felt rather like saying 'my name is Boris and I'm an alcoholic', as though it were something a little shameful: don't be different, don't make a fuss.

And then I thought two things at once. First, they're professional caterers and they're entirely used to dealing with many requests a lot weirder than this. Second, and much more importantly, I had nothing to be ashamed of; quite the opposite.

This is the third Bluffer's Guide I've written, after *The Bluffer's Guide to Brexit* and *The Bluffer's Guide to Christmas*. They're invariably great fun to work on, but with the best will in the world I never expected that doing one would be life-changing. This book really has been. I always hope that people enjoy reading *Bluffer's Guides* as much as I enjoy writing them, but this time there's a little more to it than that. This time, I hope it changes even one reader's life the way it has mine.

ALPHABET BLACK BEAN SOUP: A VEGAN GLOSSARY

Ag-gag Proposed or actual laws used to stop animal rights activists from filming inside factory farms and slaughterhouses.

AI Abbreviation of artificial insemination, the process of impregnating farmed animals. Not to be confused either with 'artificial intelligence' or what a Yorkshireman says when he first can't hear you and then agrees with whatever you've just said.

Albumen Egg white, commonly used in wine filtration. Vegans seek out wines which do not use albumen during manufacturing.

ALF Abbreviation of Animal Liberation Front, an extremist animal rights group. Not to be confused with Alf Garnett, Alf Tupper, or Alfa Romeo.

Alternative meat Vegan products designed to mimic the appearance and taste of meat.

Anthropocentrism The belief that humans are the

pinnacle of evolution, the rightful owners of everything on earth, and the appropriate yardstick by which the lives of other animals can be measured. Also a mouthful.

Apologist How radical or uncompromising vegans describe their fellow vegans who refuse to condemn non-vegans' behaviour. (Non-vegans may in turn choose to describe vegans who use the word 'apologist' as 'judgemental pricks'.)

Avocado Vegan superfood full of excellent nutrients. Staple diet of supermodels. Avocado production in Mexico, which supplies 45% of the world market, is increasingly controlled by gangs branching out from narcotics.

Backyard eggs Eggs which come from chickens which are kept in people's gardens and therefore are genuinely free range. Most vegans will still not eat these, but some think it's OK particularly in animal welfare terms when they can see with their own eyes that the hens are well treated.

Bacon troll People who troll vegan posts on social media or in online forums with remarks extolling the deliciousness of bacon or GIFs of bacon sizzling in a pan. The words 'get a life' spring to mind.

Battery cage Cages in which layer hens are crammed in with an area around the size of an iPad each to call their own. Nothing to do with either assault and battery or those bargain brands of battery called 'XtraLonglife' you get for £2 a pack in the garage, which conk out after roughly 25 minutes' use.

Big Ag The collective noun for all large food companies, implicitly referencing their economic power and political influence. Not to be confused with any statuesque ladies named Agnes.

Broiler Chicken raised to be killed for its meat.

Bycatch Fish and other marine animals killed by being unintentionally caught in nets. The word 'unintentionally' is doing some seriously heavy lifting here, as the way in which large-scale commercial fishing is conducted means that bycatch is pretty much unavoidable. From the same school of linguistic circumlocution as 'collateral damage' to describe innocent civilians killed by bombs aimed at military or government targets.

CAFO Concentrated Animal Feeding Operation. How the US Environmental Protection Agency likes to refer to factory farms.

Carcinogen Substance which can cause cancer. Two such substances are processed meat and red meat, according to the WHO (the World Health Organisation, that is, not the time-travelling Doctor or the rock band fronted by Roger Daltrey).

Carnism From a vegan's point of view, the mindset of seeing meat-eating as normal rather than a deliberate choice. Not to be confused with Kim Carnes, 1980s chanteuse best known for 'Bette Davis Eyes'. No word yet on whether Kim Carnes is a vegan (or even whether Bette Davis was).

Clean meat Meat grown in laboratories from animal cells.

EU Emissions Trading System A market based measure where participants monitor and report their emissions and surrender sufficient emission allowances to cover their reported emissions each year. Clear on that?

Factory farming Mass-breeding animals and keeping them in cramped, confined, distressing and unclean conditions.

Flexitarian Part-time vegan/vegetarian. May or may not be flexible, yoga-style.

Free range 99% of the time, distinguished by being neither 'free' nor 'range' in any commonly accepted definition of either word.

Halal Islamic term meaning 'permissible', and referring to the slaughter of an animal by slitting the throat without prior stunning.

Influencer Social media personality who has the clout to change people's lifestyles. Not to be confused with. ...

Influenza A nasty cold or an animal-transferred pandemic capable of killing millions.

Instagram Photograph-based social media site. Host to more photos of food than you ever thought possible. There may even be more food photos here than there are grains of sand on the beaches of the world or atoms in the universe.

Kosher Food conforming to Jewish dietary regulations. As with halal, the animal has its throat cut without prior stunning.

Layer Chicken bred to lay eggs.

Methane Produced by cows after eating grass and humans after eating lentils. Or mung beans.

Ocean deadzones Maritime areas depleted of marine life due to overfishing.

Outreach Vegans speaking about veganism to non-vegans in a public arena. Leafleting, stalls, fairs and so on are all examples of outreach.

Ovo-lacto Prepared to consume eggs and milk. In dietary terms, the single biggest difference between vegans and vegetarians.

Pescatarian Fish-eater. Sometimes claims to be vegetarian, but clearly isn't as, well, a fish isn't a vegetable, is it?

PETA People for the Ethical Treatment of Animals. Animal rights pressure group. Not to be confused with Blue Peter, Peter Capaldi, Peter Gabriel, Peter Parker, Peter Purves, Peter Rabbit, Struwwelpeter.

Plant Either the source of all vegan food, or an undercover police officer infiltrating animal rights groups.

Plant-based A diet which does not contain any animal products. Largely but not totally synonymous with veganism; someone who eats only vegan food but still uses non-vegan household products, buys non-vegan clothes and goes to zoos would be considered 'plant-based' rather than fully 'vegan' by most vegans.

Raw veganism Prefer to consume raw plant foods rather than cooked ones.

Seitan High protein meat-replica substance made from wheat gluten. A mainstay of vegan cuisine. Also the deity to which vegan devil-worshippers pray.

Soyboy Insult aimed at vegan men for being less masculine than their meat-eating counterparts. Humorously reclaimed by vegan men as a source of pride.

Speciesism. The view that one species is superior to another: not merely between humans and animals, but between different species of animal too (for example, considering dogs as superior to pigs). The only known species which is entirely speciesist are cats. Every single cat in the world clearly considers themselves better than any other animal out there, humans included (see *The Bluffer's Guide to Cats* for confirmation).

Trophy hunting Hunting animals not for food but for the thrill of it (and the chance to post pictures on social media, which can in some cases backfire. Unlike the gun in question, sadly).

Veganuary Scheme under which people go vegan for the month of January as a trial period. Part of the increasing annexation of months for good causes: Stoptober, Movember, Decembeard.

WFPB 'Whole-foods plant-based', where foods must be both unprocessed and vegan, such as beans, fruits, lentils, nuts, seeds, vegetables and whole grains.

Zero grazing Cattle kept permanently inside and not allowed out to graze naturally.

A BIT MORE BLUFFING...